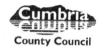

County Council

Libraries, books and more...........

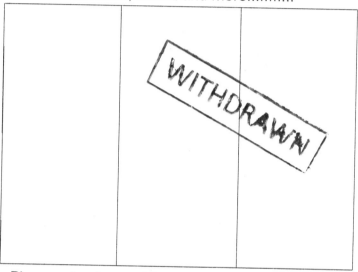

Please return/renew this item by the last date shown.
Library items may also be renewed by phone on
030 33 33 1234 (24hours) or via our website

www.cumbria.gov.uk/libraries

Cumbria Libraries

CLIC

Interactive Catalogue

Ask for a CLIC password

Independence Educational Publishers

First published by Independence Educational Publishers

The Studio, High Green

Great Shelford

Cambridge CB22 5EG

England

© Independence 2019

Copyright

Photocopy licence

ISBN-13: 978 1 86168 802 6

Printed in Great Britain

Zenith Print Group

Contents

Introduction

MENTAL HEALTH is Volume 346 in the **ISSUES** series. The aim of the series is to offer current, diverse information about important issues in our world, from a UK perspective.

ABOUT MENTAL HEALTH

Discussion around mental health issues has become more open and honest in recent years. Public figures coming forward and revealing their struggles with mental health, from pop stars to the Royal Family, has had a positive effect in destigmatising the issue and bringing it into the mainstream. However, while the number of young people reporting mental distress is on the rise, mental health services are struggling to cope with demand. This book looks at the current mental health crisis and associated issues, particularly in relation to young people.

OUR SOURCES

Titles in the **ISSUES** series are designed to function as educational resource books, providing a balanced overview of a specific subject.

The information in our books is comprised of facts, articles and opinions from many different sources, including:

⇨ Newspaper reports and opinion pieces

⇨ Website factsheets

⇨ Magazine and journal articles

⇨ Statistics and surveys

⇨ Government reports

⇨ Literature from special interest groups.

A NOTE ON CRITICAL EVALUATION

Because the information reprinted here is from a number of different sources, readers should bear in mind the origin of the text and whether the source is likely to have a particular bias when presenting information (or when conducting their research). It is hoped that, as you read about the many aspects of the issues explored in this book, you will critically evaluate the information presented.

It is important that you decide whether you are being presented with facts or opinions. Does the writer give a biased or unbiased report? If an opinion is being expressed, do you agree with the writer? Is there potential bias to the 'facts' or statistics behind an article?

ASSIGNMENTS

In the back of this book, you will find a selection of assignments designed to help you engage with the articles you have been reading and to explore your own opinions. Some tasks will take longer than others and there is a mixture of design, writing and research-based activities that you can complete alone or in a group.

FURTHER RESEARCH

At the end of each article we have listed its source and a website that you can visit if you would like to conduct your own research. Please remember to critically evaluate any sources that you consult and consider whether the information you are viewing is accurate and unbiased.

Useful weblinks

www.bma.org.uk

www.cam.ac.uk

www.england.nhs.uk

www.fullfact.org

www.gov.uk

www.headstogether.org.uk

www.independent.co.uk

www.inews.co.uk

www.mentalhealth.org.uk

www.mentalhealthtoday.co.uk

www.mentallyhealthyschools.org.uk

www.mind.org.uk

www.natcen.ac.uk

www.nhs.uk

www.open.edu

www.rethink.org

www.samaritans.org

www.sportengland.org

www.telegraph.co.uk

www.theconversation.com

www.theguardian.com

www.time-to-change.org.uk

Mental health problems – an introduction

There are many different mental health problems. Some of them have similar symptoms, so you may experience the symptoms of more than one mental health problem, or be given several diagnoses at once. Or you might not have any particular diagnosis, but still be finding things very difficult. Everyone's experience is different and can change at different times.

What types are there?

Depression

Depression is a feeling of low mood that lasts for a long time and affects your everyday life. It can make you feel hopeless, despairing, guilty, worthless, unmotivated and exhausted. It can affect your self-esteem, sleep, appetite, sex drive and your physical health.

In its mildest form, depression doesn't stop you leading a normal life, but it makes everything harder to do and seem less worthwhile. At its most severe, depression can make you feel suicidal, and be life-threatening.

Some types occur during or after pregnancy (antenatal and postnatal depression), or may come back each year around the same time (seasonal affective disorder).

Anxiety problems

Anxiety is what we feel when we are worried, tense or afraid – particularly about things that are about to happen, or which we think could happen in the future.

Occasional anxiety is a normal human experience. But if your feelings of anxiety are very strong, or last for a long time, they can be overwhelming. You might also experience physical symptoms such as sleep problems and panic attacks.

You might be diagnosed with a particular anxiety disorder, such as generalised anxiety disorder (GAD), social anxiety (social phobia), panic disorder or post-traumatic stress disorder (PTSD). But it's also possible to experience problems with anxiety without having a specific diagnosis.

Phobias

A phobia is an extreme form of fear or anxiety triggered by a particular situation (such as going outside) or object (such as spiders), even when it's very unlikely to be dangerous.

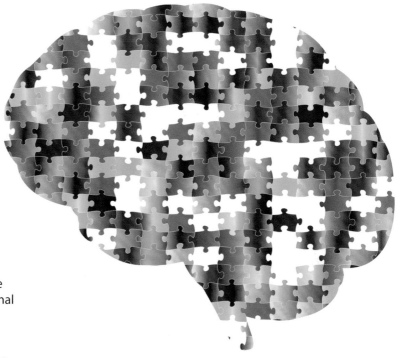

A fear becomes a phobia if the fear is out of proportion to the danger, it lasts for more than six months, and has a significant impact on how you live your day-to-day life.

Eating problems

Eating problems are not just about food. They can be about difficult things and painful feelings which you may be finding hard to face or resolve. Lots of people think that if you have an eating problem you will be over- or underweight, and that being a certain weight is always associated with a specific eating problem, but this is a myth. Anyone, regardless of age, gender or weight, can be affected by eating problems.

The most common eating disorder diagnoses are anorexia, bulimia, binge eating disorder, and other specified feeding or eating disorder (OSFED). But it's also possible to have a very difficult relationship with food and not fit the criteria for any specific diagnosis.

Obsessive-compulsive disorder (OCD)

Obsessive-compulsive disorder is a type of anxiety disorder. The term is often misused in daily conversation – for example, you might hear people talk about being 'a bit OCD', if they like things to be neat and tidy. But the reality of this disorder is a lot more complex and serious.

OCD has two main parts: obsessions (unwelcome thoughts, images, urges, worries or doubts that repeatedly appear in your mind; and compulsions (repetitive activities that you feel you have to do to reduce the anxiety caused by the obsession).

Bipolar disorder

Bipolar disorder (once called manic depression) mainly affects your mood. With this diagnosis you are likely to have times when you experience: manic or hypomanic episodes (feeling high); depressive episodes (feeling low); and potentially some psychotic symptoms.

Everyone has variations in their mood, but in bipolar disorder these swings can feel very extreme and have a big impact on your life. In between, you might have stable times where you experience fewer symptoms.

Schizophrenia

Views on schizophrenia have changed over the years. Lots of people question whether it's really a distinct condition, or actually a few different conditions that overlap. But you may still be given this diagnosis if you experience symptoms such as:

- psychosis (such as hallucinations or delusions)
- disorganised thinking and speech
- feeling disconnected from your feelings
- difficulty concentrating
- wanting to avoid people

- a lack of interest in things
- not wanting to look after yourself.

Because psychiatric experts disagree about what schizophrenia is, some people argue that this term shouldn't be used at all. Others think the name of the condition doesn't matter, and prefer to just focus on helping you manage your symptoms and meeting your individual needs.

Personality disorders

Personality disorder is a type of mental health problem where your attitudes, beliefs and behaviours cause you longstanding problems in your life. If you have this diagnosis it doesn't mean that you're fundamentally different from other people – but you may regularly experience difficulties with how you think about yourself and others, and find it very difficult to change these unwanted patterns.

There are several different categories and types of personality disorder, but most people who are diagnosed with a particular personality disorder don't fit any single category very clearly or consistently. Also, the term 'personality disorder' can sound very judgemental.

Because of this it is a particularly controversial diagnosis. Some psychiatrists disagree with using it. And many people who are given this label find it more helpful to explain their experiences in other way.

This information was published in October 2017 – to be revised in 2020.

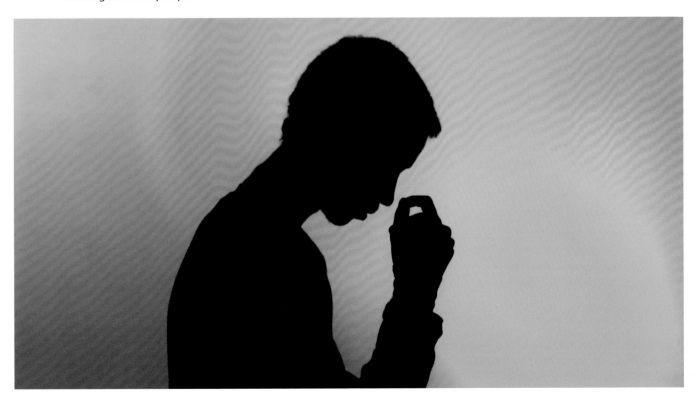

What's mental health?

The World Health Organization defines mental health as a state of wellbeing in which every individual achieves their potential, copes with the normal stresses of life, works productively and fruitfully, and is able to make a contribution to their community. Mental health includes our emotional, psychological and social wellbeing. It affects how we think, feel and act. Like physical health, mental health is something we all have. It can range across a spectrum from healthy to unwell; it can fluctuate on a daily basis and change over time.

Mental health spectrum

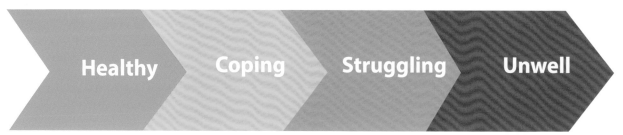

Healthy — Coping — Struggling — Unwell

Adapted from Centre for Mental Health

Good mental health helps children:

- learn and explore the world
- feel, express and manage a range of positive and negative emotions
- form and maintain good relationships with others
- cope with, and manage change and uncertainty
- develop and thrive.

Building strong mental health early in life can help children build their self-esteem, learn to settle themselves and engage positively with their education. This, in turn, can lead to improved academic attainment, enhanced future employment opportunities and positive life choices.

Promoting mental health

There is good evidence that schools can help all children develop essential social and emotional skills through delivering bespoke sessions designed to cultivate these skills, through ensuring broader opportunities are capitalised on to reinforce skills across the curriculum and through whole-school modelling of these skills. Social and emotional skills prevent poor mental health from developing, help all children cope effectively with setbacks and remain healthy. These whole-school programmes are noted to benefit all children but particularly those who are at most risk.

Schools can support these children by providing them with additional help to understand and manage their thoughts, feelings and behaviour and build skills that help them to thrive, such as working in a team, persistence and self-awareness.

Coping skills

Mental health doesn't mean being happy all the time. Neither does it mean avoiding stress altogether. Coping and adjusting to setbacks are critical life skills for children, but it's important that they develop positive, rather than negative, coping skills.

Negative coping skills are attitudes and behaviours that have often been learned in the absence of positive support and in the face of stressful and often traumatic events and experiences which, over time, may put good mental health at risk.

Example: children at risk of or experiencing maltreatment in the home may have learned to react quickly and in a certain way (flight or fight or freeze) to survive and keep themselves safe. But in a classroom, these reactions may not work well and could get them into trouble, disrupt learning and make them unpopular with teachers and peers. In the longer term, these learned behaviours may also impact on their mental health and wellbeing, sense of belonging, educational achievements, peer relationships and life chances.

Positive coping skills are ways of thinking, attitudes and behaviours that allow children to deal with stress or adversity and which help them flourish. These positive coping skills form an important part of a child's ability to be resilient in the face of setbacks and challenges. Children who have cultivated robust coping skills can still thrive with support, even when they are mentally unwell.

What affects child mental health?

A child's mental health is influenced by many things over time. Children have different personalities and they will be exposed to a range of factors in their homes and communities that can trigger worsening mental health (risk factors), or alternatively protect them and help them feel able to cope (protective factors). Ideally, all children should have at least one adult in their life who is monitoring whether they are coping or not.

Identifying children who are struggling

Deteriorating mental health is not always easy to spot and can be overlooked until things reach crisis point. At least two children in every primary school class (based on average class size of 27) are likely to have a diagnosable mental health condition. This rises to three to four students in every class by secondary school age (Green, 2005).[1] Around a further six to eight children in each primary school class will be struggling just below this 'unwell' threshold (Wyn, J. et al., 2000).[2]

Mental health: why it's important to schools

Schools are the ideal environment in which to promote and support the mental health of primary age children, ensuring they can reach their potential and take advantage of opportunities throughout their lives:

- Most children spend a significant amount of time in school and school staff are in a good position to piece together the jigsaw of what may be undermining a child's mental health.

- Parents also tend to approach schools first for advice when children experience mental health challenges.

- There is strong evidence that school programmes which promote social and emotional skills can improve mental health and academic attainment.

- Children with good mental health are more positive, settled and can achieve better academically.

- Early help can also prevent unnecessary crises, poor life chances and significant costs affecting the public purse.

February 2018

[1] Green, H., McGinnity, A., Meltzer, H., Ford, T. & Goodman, R. (2005). The mental health of children and young people in Great Britain 2004. Basingstoke, Hampshire: Palgrave.

[2] Wyn, J. et al., 2000. MindMatters, a whole school approach promoting mental health and wellbeing. *Australian and New Zealand Journal of Psychiatry*, 34(4), pp. 594–60.

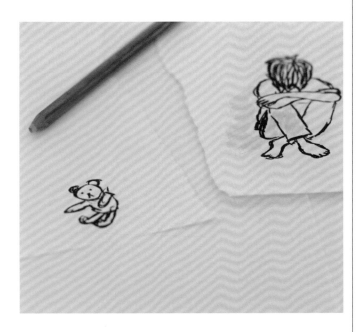

Do I have mental health problems and should I get some help?

Chances are that within your lifetime you will experience some form of mental health problem, the most common of these being depression and anxiety. But because most people with a mental health condition will never access any formal types of support or treatment, many of these mental health problems will go undiagnosed. Longitudinal studies (i.e. research conducted with the same people over many years) support the notion that experiencing a diagnosable mental health condition or disorder at some stage during a person's life is the norm, not the exception. A study recently published by Schaefer and colleagues (2017) established that over 80% of participants from their health and development study were found to have a diagnosable mental health condition, from the time of their birth to midlife. This was amongst a representative group of more than 1,000 people studied over a four-decade period.

So if most of us will experience mental ill-health at some time in our lives, why is it so hard for people to recognise the signs and symptoms of this in themselves, and subsequently access treatment? Here are five reasons why people may be reluctant to seek professional help:

1: Mental health stigma and its impact

Regrettably there is still a stigma associated with being diagnosed with a mental health condition. Understandably, given this stigma, people with mental health problems can worry that they will get judged and seen as weak, so many can end up keeping their experiences to themselves or denying that their problems exist. Fortunately, there is now greater protection against discrimination on the basis of mental ill-health, as a result of legislation like the 2010 Equality Act. This legal protection makes it easier for people to open up about their mental health problems, especially in the workplace. In addition to this legal advancement, large-scale public campaigns have sought to challenge mental health stigma, and increase awareness of its negative impact. For example 'Time to Change' in England, which has sought to reduce mental health-related stigma and discrimination since 2009.

2: Problems in the mild to moderate range

Every individual is different, and it can be hard for us to recognise if what we are experiencing is 'normal' or not. As the saying goes, 'normal is nothing more than a cycle on a washing machine' and the real norm is that most of us will experience a period of mental ill-health sometime in our lives. For the majority this will take the form of something in the 'mild to moderate range' of difficulties. For example, temporary periods of feeling low are common, and are often a normal reaction to the stressors we can experience. For most people, seeking support from their friends and/or family members can help them get through these difficult times. Self-help resources and interventions like mindfulness can also be useful in assisting people in overcoming life's challenges. If your low mood or other mental health problems persist, affecting your sleep, relationships, job and/or appetite, this can indicate that you may require some additional help, and a visit to your general practitioner (GP) would be recommended.

> *"Normal is nothing more than a cycle on a washing machine."*
> *– Whoopi Goldberg*

3: When is it really bad?

It is important to be able to recognise when a mental health problem has progressed to becoming a major issue. Many people can struggle to notice in themselves when their mental health problems are more severe. This might seem surprising, but because a person can be suffering over a long period of time, their symptoms may not initially have a dramatic impact. In addition to this, even when mental health problems can be debilitating, a person may still feel that their problems aren't bad enough to warrant professional treatment. If you are having persistent worries, distressing feelings or frightening experiences it can really help to get support and information. This may initially involve visiting your GP. Sometimes people may need specialised mental health services and a GP can help people access services. GPs assist many people with their mental health problems, and recently there have been some indications that they are supporting more and more people with mental health problems.

4: Securing treatment

There are a range of supports and interventions available for people with mental health problems. But it can be hard to know what to look for when attempting to get help. It can be overwhelming and exhausting just finding the right type of support for you. Do you want a psychotherapist? A practitioner psychologist? A counsellor? Is medication an option? Is a combination of medication and face-to-face therapy the best interventions for you? What is funded and what do you need to pay for yourself? There

are also the challenges associated with getting a session or appointment that is at a time and place that is convenient to you. There is Improving Access to Psychological Therapies (IAPT), which began almost 10 years ago and has delivered treatment to over 900,000 adults with anxiety and depression, both in individual sessions and in group-based format. However, there can be waiting lists for IAPT and for other state-funded forms of therapy. For those with the funds available to pay for treatment, websites like welldoing.org can assist people to find a therapist.

5: A lack of hope

Hope is of fundamental importance to all humans, but when someone is struggling with mental health problems, this can be compromised. Sometimes people will not access help, even if they recognise that they have significant issues, in part because they feel so negatively about their future. A lack of hope in regard to one's future is a sign that a person needs to seek help. It could be from a family member, your GP, the Samaritans, from the MIND infoline or a trusted friend.

December 2017

Schaefer, J. D. et al. (2017). Enduring mental health: Prevalence and prediction. *Journal of Abnormal Psychology*, 126(2), 212–224.

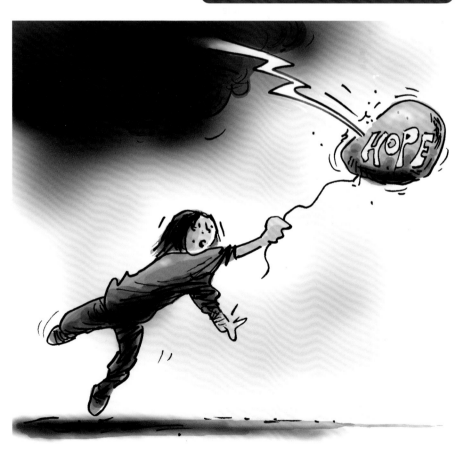

Reporting on mental health

An extract from Time to Change's media guidelines.

If you are tasked with covering a story involving somebody who you believe may have a mental health problem, here are a few things to consider:

- Is it relevant to the story that the featured person has a mental illness?

- Don't speculate about someone's mental health being a factor in the story unless you know this to be 100% true.

- Don't provide an 'on air' diagnosis or encourage 'experts' to do so.

- Is it appropriate for the person's mental illness to be mentioned in the headline or lead?

- Who are your sources? Can you rely on eyewitnesses or neighbours to provide facts or has an assumption been made about someone's mental health status?

- Include contextualising facts. Remember people with severe mental illnesses are more likely to be victims – rather than perpetrators – of violent crime.

- Consider consulting people with mental health problems as part of your research, not just as case studies. They are experts on their own conditions.

Language

Choosing the right language to describe people with mental health problems is important. Using inaccurate terms can reinforce stereotypes and stigma. Here are the most common misused words, as well as some alternative suggestions.

Avoid using	Instead try	Why?
'unhinged', 'maniac', 'loony' or 'mad'.	'a person with a mental health problem'.	These words are usually linked to dangerousness or strange behaviour.
'a psycho' or 'a schizo'.	A person who has experienced psychosis or 'a person with schizophrenia'.	Linked to popular culture and dangerousness. Beware of using as a blanket description for mental health problems.
'a schizophrenic' or 'a depressive'.	Someone who 'has a diagnosis of', 'currently experiencing' or 'is being treated for…'.	People are more than their illness, it doesn't define them.
'the mentally ill', a 'victim', 'the afflicted', 'a person suffering from', 'a sufferer'.	'people with mental health problems'.	Many people with mental health problems live full lives and many also recover.
'prisoners' or 'inmates' (in a psychiatric hospital).	'mental health patients', 'patients', 'service users' or 'clients'.	People are treated in hospital not locked away in prison.
'released' (from a hospital).	'discharged'.	Same as someone with a physical health problem.
'happy pills'.	'antidepressants' 'medication' or 'prescription drugs'.	Undermines the possible impact of depression suggests a 'quick fix'.

Other common language mistakes

- 'Schizophrenic' or 'bipolar' should not be used to mean 'two minds' or a 'split personality' OR be used metaphorically to describe something with two different sides.

- Somebody who is angry is not 'psychotic'.

- A person who is down or unhappy is not the same as someone experiencing clinical depression.

April 2017

MENTAL HEALTH IN THE UK:
The big picture

Adapted from the Mental Health Foundation's *Managing Mental Health in the Workplace* e-book

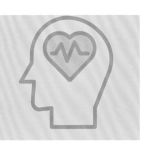

TODAY

9 out of **10**

people with mental health problems experience stigma and discrimination

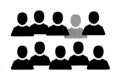

Anxiety and depression is the most common mental problem

At least

1 in **4**

people will experience some kind of mental health problem each year

THE GENDER DIVIDE

37%

of men are feeling worried or low. Yet their wives, partners, other relatives and friends may have no idea there's a problem

Women are between 20 and 40% more likely than men to develop a mental health problem

Since 1981, the proportion of male to female suicides has increased steadily with

4 in **5** suicides being male

Half of women with perinatal mental health problems are not identified or treated costing the UK an estimated

£8.1bn

THE COST TO UK BUSINESSES

1 in **5**

people take a day off work due to stress

In the last 6 years the number of working days lost to stress depression and anxiety has **increased by 24%**

70 million

working days are lost each year due to mental ill health, costing Britain annually **£70–100bn.**

Presenteeism can **double the cost**

Around **£££££££**

£1 in every £8 spent

on long-term physical conditions is linked to **poor mental health and wellbeing**

Less than half of employees said they would feel able to talk openly with their line manager if they were suffering from stress

A quarter of people consider resigning due to stress

In a survey of UK adults

56%

said they **would not hire someone with depression** even if they were the best candidate for the job

AROUND THE COUNTRY

The UK has the fourth highest rate of antidepressant prescriptions in Europe at

50m

per year

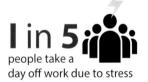

In Scotland, nearly **1 in 10** adults had two or more symptoms of depression or anxiety in 2012/13

The North East has the highest suicide rate in England while London has the lowest

Prevalence of mental illness in Northern Ireland is 25% higher than in England

People in Liverpool were rated as the most anxious with an anxiety score of nearly **30%**

Aberystwyth and Coventry were rated as having the least happy employees

Wolverhampton were lowest at around **10%**

Sources: NHS Information Centre for Health and Social Care | NICE Common mental health disorders | Time to Change | Mind | The King's Fund & Centre for Mental Health | 2014 CMO annual report: public mental health |Business in the Community 2014 | Daniel Freeman – Oxford University | Office for National Statistics | NHS figures 2014 | Conference Genie | Health and Safety Executive | Centre Forum Atlas of Variation | Scottish Health Survey 2013 | Centre for Mental Health 2014, London | Action Mental Health Northern Ireland| Mind & Chartered Institute of Personnel Development 2011 | London School of Economics & Political Sciences

We need to rethink how we classify mental illness

Psychiatric diagnosis must serve an ethical purpose: relieving certain forms of suffering and disease. Science alone can't do that.

By Tamara Kayali Browne

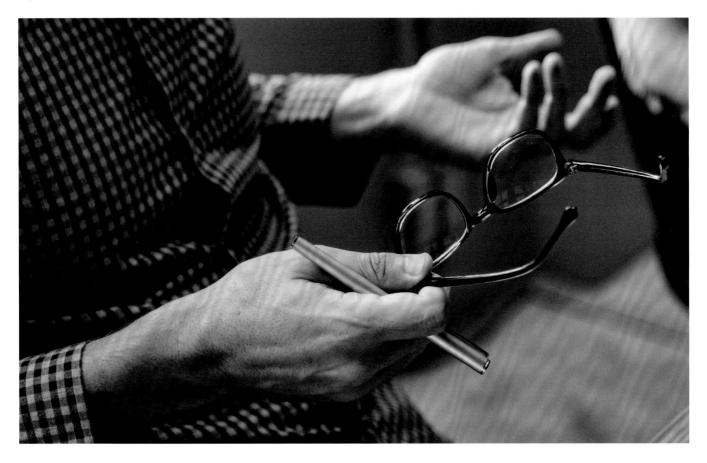

How do we decide what emotions, thoughts and behaviours are normal, abnormal or pathological? This is essentially what a select group of psychiatrists decide each time they revise the Diagnostic and Statistical Manual of Mental Disorders (DSM), considered a 'bible' for mental health professionals worldwide.

But questions like this cannot be answered by scientists alone. This was famously demonstrated when homosexuality was declassified as a mental illness in the DSM in 1973. The decision was not based on new scientific evidence but came about due to pressure from activists. Cases such as this show the limitations of psychiatry and is where I believe philosophers, sociologists and ethicists could be of use.

The DSM was first published by the American Psychiatric Association in 1952 to create a common language and standard criteria for the way we classify mental disorders. It's now used around the world by clinicians, researchers, insurance and pharmaceutical companies, the legal system, health regulators and policy makers, to name a few.

Now in its fifth edition, revisions have gradually expanded the number of mental disorders, while also removing some

as understanding or values change. Over the years, many of these amendments have courted controversy.

These days, criticisms of the DSM are that it medicalises normal behaviour such as fidgetiness, noisiness and shyness.

Currently, three temper tantrums a week, negativity, irritability and anger would qualify a child to be labelled with disruptive mood dysregulation disorder. The label assumes first that the child is suffering from a problem, and second that the problem is pathological. Yet one may also question why it is the child who must be labelled and not the parents. For example, why do we not have a diagnosis called inability to discipline one's child disorder?

What the 'problem' is and who is judged to be the party 'suffering' from it are value judgments which carry with them the cultural biases and assumptions of the individuals making those judgments. If we don't examine value judgements properly, we risk making judgements that are discriminatory or harmful.

For example, hysteria was mental disorder that supposedly only affected women and included a wide range of 'symptoms' such as emotional outbursts, hallucinations, too much or too little sexual appetite, irritability and trouble-making. Although hysteria has now disappeared from official psychiatric diagnosis, there are elements of it present within other psychiatric diagnoses, most notably premenstrual dysphoric disorder (PMDD).

Commonly described as a more severe form of premenstrual stress (PMS), PMDD has been accused of labelling as a mental disorder normal and understandable reactions to the sort of stressful circumstances that disproportionately affect women in a modern society that still has not achieved gender equality.

In this way, psychiatric diagnosis could act as a way of brushing aside indicators of social injustices.

Likewise, sadness and changes in sleep, eating and so on can be normal and understandable reactions to loss (e.g. in the case of bereavement), not necessarily indicators of mental illness. In fact, behaviours like these can act as a positive sign that something is wrong, functioning as a catalyst for changing one's situation for the better.

But the DSM only focuses on these 'symptoms' and does not take into account the individual's context. This in itself is a value judgement.

This is why our process of classifying mental illnesses should involve experts for whom examining value judgements is their bread and butter – philosophers. Bioethicists and philosophers of psychiatry are trained in bringing value judgements to light and analysing them in depth.

The way we classify mental illnesses also has broad implications for those diagnosed and for society – something that sociologists would be well placed to consider.

We could make good use of these experts by requiring each revision of the DSM to pass through an ethics assessment by an independent panel made up of philosophers, sociologists and ethicists.

Philosophers could identify and deliberate the value issues, sociologists could present the possible social consequences of proposed changes, and ethicists could make the complex harm/benefit analyses and ethical trade-offs that will inevitably be involved.

The panel also needs to have 'teeth', so it should have the power to veto or modify a category.

This might sound like a provocative proposal, but it is similar to the procedure we already have for scientific studies. Just as these studies must gain ethics approval before they go ahead in order to mitigate harm to participants and the community, having an ethics review panel would be an extra step of 'checks and balances' for the DSM.

While those involved in making the DSM come from a variety of backgrounds – primarily psychiatrists, psychologists, social workers and clinicians – none have been primarily ethicists or philosophers.

And while some psychiatrists might have the training and experience that enables them to examine value judgements, it would be unreasonable to expect that to be the case, just as it would be unreasonable to expect ethicists and philosophers to be able to evaluate scientific judgements.

The solution I propose is based on the idea that psychiatric diagnosis should serve an ethical purpose – relieving certain forms of suffering and disease.

In light of this ethical purpose, we must do our utmost to consider value judgements that can cloud our view of 'illness' and how it should be treated. I believe establishing an ethics review panel for the DSM can go a significant way towards achieving that goal.

30 October 2017

Dr Tamara Kayali Browne is a lecturer in health ethics at Deakin University's school of medicine. She is the author of A Role for Philosophers, Sociologists and Bioethicists in Revising the DSM: A Philosophical Case Conference, published in the journal *Philosophy, Psychiatry & Psychology.*

This article was amended on 1 November 2017 to clarify the declassification of homosexuality and hysteria.

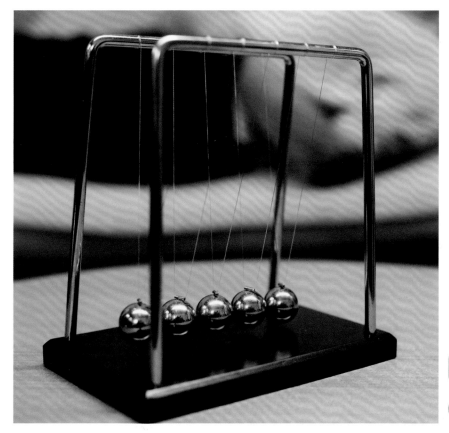

Key findings from the *2017 Mental Health of Children and Young People* report

By Franziska Marcheselli, Researcher

The *2017 Mental Health of Children and Young People* survey is our first robust update on child mental health since the last survey in 2004. This has been published by NHS Digital.

A random sample of children, their parents and teachers from across England were interviewed. While five to 15-year-olds were also interviewed in 1999 and 2004 — the latest survey provides England's first data on the prevalence of mental disorder in two to four-year-olds. It also spans into adulthood by covering 17 to 19-year-olds.

What is a mental disorder?

Most surveys use short screening instruments to identify who might have a mental disorder. This survey series is different. Mental disorders were identified using standardised diagnostic criteria from the International Classification of Diseases (ICD-10).

Disorders were grouped into four categories: emotional, behavioural, hyperactivity and other less common disorders.

While symptoms may be present in many children, to count as a disorder they had to be sufficiently severe to cause distress to the child or impair their functioning (World Health Organization, 1993).

Have things changed over time?

The prevalence of mental disorders in five to 15-year-olds (the age group covered in all surveys in this series) has increased a little over time: from 9.7% in 1999 and 10.1% in 2004, to 11.2% in 2017.

There is much stability over time in most disorder groups. However, as you can see from the chart below, emotional disorders have inched up from 4.3% in 1999 to 5.8% in 2017.

Behavioural disorders have always been the most common type in childhood (which was found in 1999 and 2004); however, this no longer seems to be the case — in 2017 emotional disorders were the most common disorder type.

Trends in different types of disorder in five to 15-year-olds, 1999 to 2017

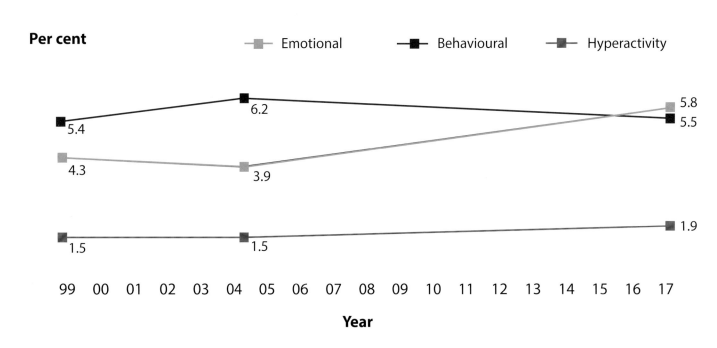

Per cent

Emotional — Behavioural — Hyperactivity

5.4 — 6.2 — 5.8 — 5.5
4.3 — 3.9
1.5 — 1.5 — 1.9

99 00 01 02 03 04 05 06 07 08 09 10 11 12 13 14 15 16 17

Year

Base: five to 19-year-olds
Per cent

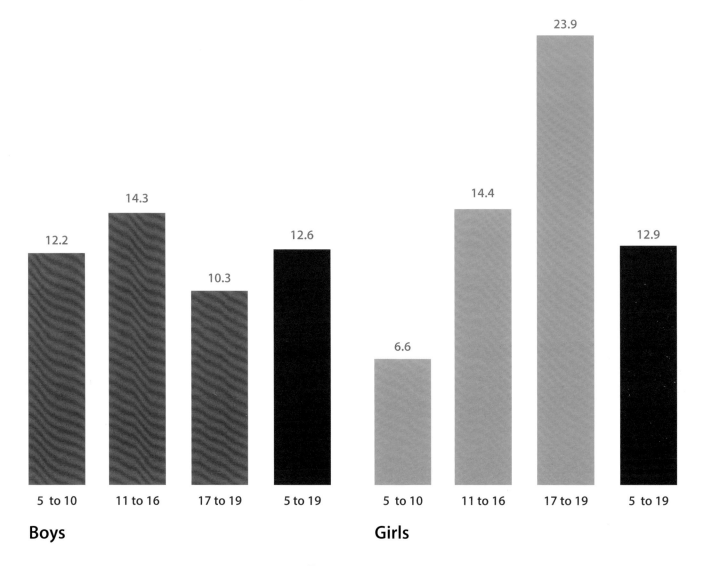

Source: NHS Digital

Age group

What did we find in 2017?

One in eight (12.8%) five to 19-year-olds had at least one mental disorder at the time of interview. One in eighteen (5.5%) preschool children (those aged two to four) were also identified with a mental disorder around the time of the interview.

In five to 19-year-olds, rates were highest in girls aged 17 to 19. Almost a quarter (23.9%) met the criteria for having at least one mental disorder.

One in 12 (8.1%) five to 19-year-olds had an emotional disorder like anxiety or depression.

This was the most common disorder type. About one in 20 (4.6%) had a behavioural disorder, about one in 50 (2.1%) had a less common disorder, such as an eating disorder or autism, and about one in 60 (1.6%) had a hyperactivity disorder.

What does this mean?

These survey findings have updated the current prevalence estimates of mental disorder in two to 19-year-olds living in England. They have shown that rates of emotional disorders have risen. The findings have highlighted older girls as a high-risk group for poor mental health, as have other studies such as the *2014 Adult Psychiatric Morbidity Survey*. There is a need to monitor this age group for whom we have less data for.

22 November 2018

1.4 million people referred to NHS mental health therapy in the past year

Over one million referrals to NHS talking therapies for depression and anxiety were made last year according to new, official data.

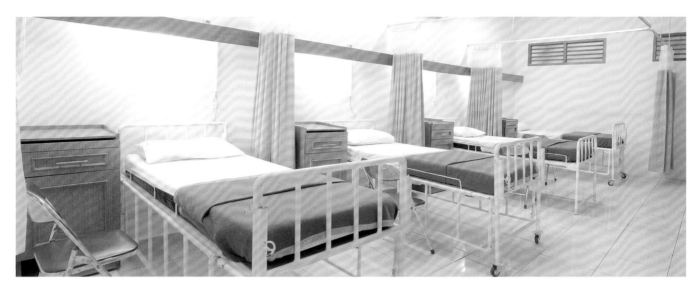

Of the 1.4 million new referrals for talking therapies as part of NHS England's Increasing Access to Talking Therapies (IAPT) programme, 965,000 people began treatment, a 32,000 rise on patient numbers from the year before.

As well as increasing numbers of people getting treatment, performance statistics for 2016/17 show that waiting times are decreasing and recovery rates improving. The number of people recovering from their condition has increased on the previous 12 months, with over 50% of patients making a recovery in every month of this year.

IAPT is a key element of NHS England's improvements to mental health services, offering talking therapies to people with common conditions including depression and anxiety. Expanding access to this type of early intervention care will mean people's conditions are spotted and treated sooner, reducing the need for more intensive, and higher cost, treatments.

The new findings come after the *New York Times* described the IAPT programme as 'the world's most ambitious effort to treat depression, anxiety and other common mental illnesses'.

Claire Murdoch, NHS England's National Director for Mental Health, said: 'Ever increasing numbers of people are getting treated by the NHS and recovering from mental ill-health.

'Talking therapists in the NHS helped nearly one million people last year, and not only are more patients getting help more quickly, but their chances of recovering, thanks to NHS support, are improving significantly.

'However, we are not complacent. Mental health services have for too long been neglected, so even with significant extra funding of more than £1 billion over five years, raising standards of care to a consistently high level will take further years of hard work and continued investment.'

The analysis of mental health services, compiled by NHS Digital, shows that:

> 567,000 people finished a course of NHS talking therapy in 2016/17: 30,000 more patients than in the year before.

> Waiting times are improving, with 88% of people waiting less than 18 weeks for treatment, and nearly nine in ten patients less than six weeks.

> As well as recovery rates improving to an average of 49% over the course of the year, 65% of patients showed 'reliable improvement' as a result of treatment.

22 December 2017

www.england.nhs.uk

Setting more exams to combat stress among school students is utterly absurd

An article from **The Conversation**

THE CONVERSATION

By Ceri Brown

Schools minister Nick Gibb reportedly advised MPs that young people should face more frequent tests in secondary school, to better prepare them for the exam stress they experience by the time they take their GCSEs. This is a surprising and somewhat shortsighted approach – not unlike proposing more regular alcohol consumption as the solution to binge drinking.

It is hard to understand what appears to be a blatant disregard for the mental health of children and young people on the part of the schools' minister – especially given that this government has repeatedly called on schools to play a larger role in addressing the purported mental health crisis among students. The prime minister herself has called for an end to the 'hidden injustice' of mental illness that 'too often starts in childhood and that when left untreated, can blight lives'.

Stressed-out students

To be clear, there is no doubt that exams contribute to mental health problems among young people. A 2015 report by the National Teachers Union concluded that:

"Children and young people are suffering from increasingly high levels of school-related anxiety and stress, disaffection and mental health problems. This is caused by increased pressure from tests/exams; greater awareness at younger ages of their own 'failure'; and the increased rigour and academic demands of the curriculum."

These findings are supported by 2009/10 survey data from the World Health Organization and findings by the children's charity ChildLine in both 2014 and 2015, which highlight that children and young people in England are suffering from growing levels of school-related anxiety and stress.

A recent survey carried out by the Association for Teachers and Lecturers (ATL) found that 82% of educators believe children and young people are under more pressure now than they were ten years ago, with 89% considering that testing and exams were the biggest cause. Some research has even drawn a link between the performance pressure created by the education system, and the development of suicidal thoughts and self-harm among young people.

Ignoring the evidence

Gibb's own colleagues on the health and education select committees have recognised the harmful effects of exam pressure, following a joint inquiry into the impacts of education on children's mental health. Perfectionism has become a harmful epidemic among young people, as they attempt to meet the demands of modern society. So to suggest more exams, as a means to combat the stress brought about by exams, misses the mark by a mile.

The schools minister denied that reforms to the curriculum were adding to the pressure on students, claiming that 'there are a raft of real-world pressures' – including social media – weighing on young people today. He didn't explain how imposing more tests could possibly alleviate those pressures. Nearly 20 years of empirical research shows us that test preparation can actually obstruct learning, contribute to anxiety and dampen motivation, for both teachers and learners. This is the ultimate absurdity in Gibb's defence of an exhausted testing system.

9 February 2018

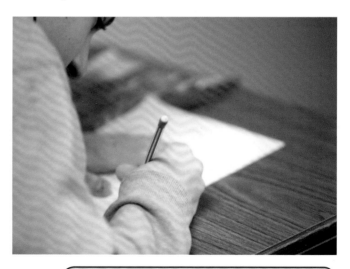

www.theconversation.com

Exam stress for school children

By Joseph O'Leary

In brief

Claim

There is a rising problem of mental stress among children because of exams.

Conclusion

There's evidence to support this from children's counselling services and the views of school leaders in England, but we don't yet know much more about how common exam stress is across the UK more generally.

"Faiza [Shaheen], do you think there is a rising problem of mental stress among children because of exams?"
David Dimbleby 15 February 2018

"It's not a matter of thinking. It's a fact, isn't it? It's just there."
Faiza Shaheen 15 February 2018

Exam stress clearly affects children in the UK, and from what we've seen there's some evidence from counselling services and school leaders that it's a growing problem.

This exchange from *BBC Question Time* comes off the back of reports that new times tables checks could be rolled out in primary schools in England.

Childline is a service that provides advice and counselling to anyone under 19 in the UK, and is part of the NSPCC. It delivered over 3,000 counselling sessions online or over the phone on exam stress in 2016/17, which is a 2% increase on what it dealt with in 2015/16 and 11% up on two years ago.

12 to 15-year-olds were the most likely to be counselled about exam stress, according to the charity, although it saw the biggest rise in contact from 16 to 18-year-olds.

As the NSPCC previously reported: 'young people told counsellors how overwhelmed they were by the whole exam process. Excessive workloads, struggling with subjects and not being prepared for exams all contributed to young people feeling stressed and anxious.'

There were also findings last year from *The Key* – which supports and provides information to school leaders. It surveyed its members, who are school leaders and governors, to find out their concerns about the state of education in England specifically.

When asked if they worried more about pupils' mental health during exams than they did two years ago, 81% of primary leaders agreed, and 78% agreed they had noticed increased stress, anxiety and panic attacks among their pupils over the same period.

This comes off the back of changes to the curriculum for schools in England in 2014.

Among other things, this introduced new and more rigorous Sats tests in 2016 for children in Year 2 (aged 6-7) and Year 6 (aged 10-11). We can't say how much these changes might have caused the increased concerns shown by school leaders in the survey.

The survey findings from *The Key* were adjusted to make them more representative of schools across England, although we don't know if there is any selection bias. We've asked *The Key* for more details about the survey.

On its own, this kind of work can only tell us so much about this issue. The figures from Childline don't tell us about children who don't come forward and use these counselling services, for example.

The Office for National Statistics (ONS) has compiled an overview of the research that's available into the mental health of young people both in England and in the UK more widely.

We also know that exams aren't the only things that are changing for children and having an impact on mental health in schools. More children using social media report having symptoms of mental ill-health, according to findings from the ONS a few years ago.

16 February 2018

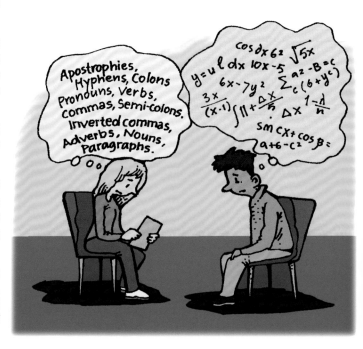

Teenagers who access mental health services see significant improvements, study shows.

The study, published in *Lancet Psychiatry*, found that 14-year-old adolescents who had contact with mental health services had a greater decrease in depressive symptoms than those with similar difficulties but without contact. By the age of 17, the odds of reporting clinical depression were more than seven times higher in individuals without contact than in service users who had been similarly depressed at baseline.

Researchers from the Department of Psychiatry recruited 1,238 14-year-old adolescents and their primary caregivers from secondary schools in Cambridgeshire, and followed them up at the age of 17. Their mental state and behaviour was assessed by trained researchers, while the teenagers self-reported their depressive symptoms. Of the participants, 126 (11%) had a current mental illness at start of the study – and only 48 (38%) of these had had contact with mental health services in the year prior to recruitment.

Contact with mental health services appeared to be of such value that after three years the levels of depressive symptoms of service users with a mental disorder were similar to those of 996 unaffected individuals.

'Mental illness can be a terrible burden on individuals, but our study shows clearly that if we intervene at an early stage, we can see potentially dramatic improvements in adolescents' symptoms of depression and reduce the risk that they go on to develop severe depressive illness,' says Sharon Neufeld, first author of the study and a research associate at in the Department of Psychiatry.

The Cambridge study is believed to be the first study in adolescents to support the role of contact with mental health services in improving mental health by late adolescence. Previous studies have reported that mental health service use has provided little or no benefit to adolescents, but the researchers argue that this may be because the design of those studies did not consider whether service users had a mental disorder or not. The approach taken on this new study enabled it to compare as closely as possible to the present study of statistically-balanced-treated versus untreated individuals with a mental disorder in a randomised control trial.

The researchers say their study highlights the need to improve access to mental health services for children and adolescents. Figures published in 2015 show that NHS spending on children's mental health services in the UK has fallen by 5.4% in real terms since 2010 to £41 million, despite an increase in demand. This has led to an increase in referrals and waiting times and an increase in severe cases that require longer stays in inpatient facilities.

On 9 January this year, the Prime Minister announced plans to transform the way we deal with mental illness in the UK at every stage of a person's life – not just in our hospitals, but in our classrooms, at work and in our communities – adding: 'This starts with ensuring that children and young people get the help and support they need and deserve – because we know that mental illness too often starts in childhood and that when left untreated, can blight lives, and become entrenched.'

Professor Ian Goodyer, who led the study, has cautiously welcomed the commitment from the Prime Minister and her Government. 'The emphasis going forward should be on early detection and intervention to help mentally-ill teens in schools, where there is now an evidence base for psychosocial intervention,' he says. 'We need to ensure, however, that there is a clear pathway for training and supervision of school-based psychological workers and strong connections to NHS child and adolescent mental health services for those teens who will need additional help.

'As always, the devil is in the detail. The funding of services and how the effectiveness of intervention is monitored will be critical if we are to reduce mental illness risks over the adolescent years. With the right measures and school-based community infrastructure, I believe this can be achieved.'

18 January 2017

The research was funded by Wellcome and the National Institute for Health Research.

Reference: Neufeld, S. et al. Reduction in adolescent depression after contact with mental health services: a longitudinal cohort study in the UK. *Lancet Psychiatry*; 10 Jan 2017; DOI: 10.1016/S2215-0366(17)30002-0

School mental health referrals rise by more than a third

By Paul Gallagher

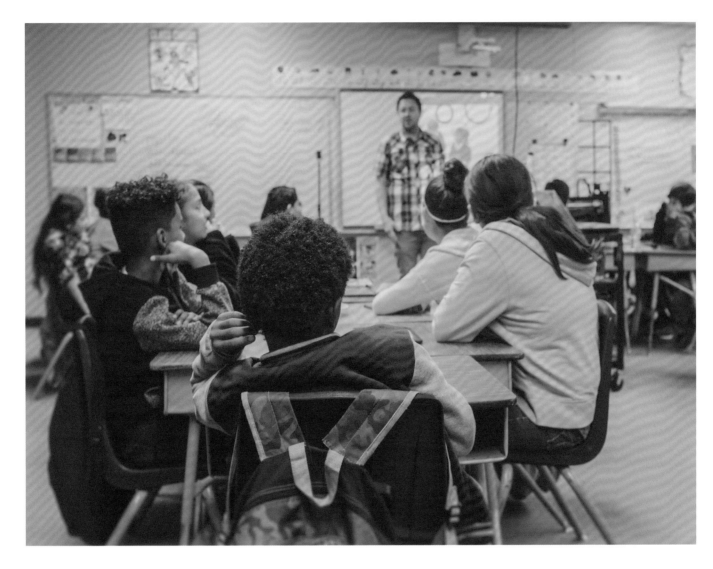

The number of referrals by schools seeking mental health treatment for troubled pupils has increased by more than a third in the last three years, the NSPCC has revealed.

The charity found schools seeking professional help for pupils from NHS Child and Adolescent Mental Health Services (CAMHS) made 123,713 referrals since 2014/15. The majority (56%) came from primary schools, which experts said could be a result of a lack of funding and services to support children in those settings.

Referrals have been steadily increasing every year, reaching 34,757 in 2017/18 – the equivalent of 183 every school day, Freedom of Information responses by NHS trusts in England to the chldren's charity reveal. The NSPCC is warning that increased demand for mental health support is placing the system under real pressure, jeopardising the wellbeing of thousands of children.

Nearly a third (31%) of referrals from schools to CAMHS over the last three years were declined treatment as they did not meet the criteria for support.

The NSPCC is now calling on the Government with their Are You There? campaign to invest some of this funding into early support services for children. Its Childline service has seen a 26% increase in the number of counselling sessions with children about mental health issues over the past four years.

Some young people have told Childline that they only received specialist support when they reached crisis point, and have even asked Childline counsellors to act on their behalf to get help quicker.

Waiting lists

One 17-year-old girl told Childline: 'I suffer with anxiety and panic attacks and find it difficult to leave the house or get out of bed. I was referred to CAMHS but I was on a waiting list for eight months and during that time my anxiety got worse so I never went because I was too scared.'

Last week, a damning select committee report found that the Government's £300 million plans to improve mental health provision for children 'lacks ambition and will provide no help to the majority of children who desperately need it'. The NSPCC is calling on government to increase the amount of funding it gives to Childline, to ensure it can reach even more children who are struggling.

Peter Wanless, NSPCC chief executive, said: 'We have seen a marked increase in counselling about mental health, and fully expect it to continue. It is vital that government urgently provides more funding to Childline and help children who don't have access to support elsewhere.'

Dr Max Davie, from the Royal College of Paediatrics and Child Health, said: 'Paediatricians working in the community have also noted a surge in referrals for emotional and behavioural difficulties, often once CAMHS have rejected the referral. As professionals who work closely with local authorities we are aware of widespread cuts to behavioural support in the educational sector, leaving schools exposed and unsupported.'

and technology and social media. The report found work-related stress in NHS staff has reached 'alarming levels'.

Recent figures show that in 2016, 15 million working days were lost because of stress, anxiety or depression. Frontline healthcare staff in the NHS, particularly those supporting clinical staff, ambulance staff and nurses have the highest absence rates.

Mental Health Foundation director Isabella Goldie called for the introduction of 'well-being days' for public sector workers. 'Stress is one of the great public health challenges of our time, but it still isn't being taken as seriously as physical health concerns,' she said.

14 May 2018

Stressed nation

Meanwhile, three-quarters of people in the UK have felt 'overwhelmed or unable to cope' at some point in the last year, according to the largest study of its kind. Young people are most likely to be highly stressed with 83% of 18-24-year-olds saying this compared to 65% of people aged 55 and over. A gender divide also emerged: 81% of women felt this way compared to 67% of men. The survey of 4,619 people, commissioned by the Mental Health Foundation for its *Stress – Are We Coping?* report, also found that almost a third of people (32%) had experienced suicidal thoughts or feelings because of stress. Meanwhile one in six people (16%) said they had self-harmed as a result of feelings of stress.

The most likely causes are long-term health conditions, work, money

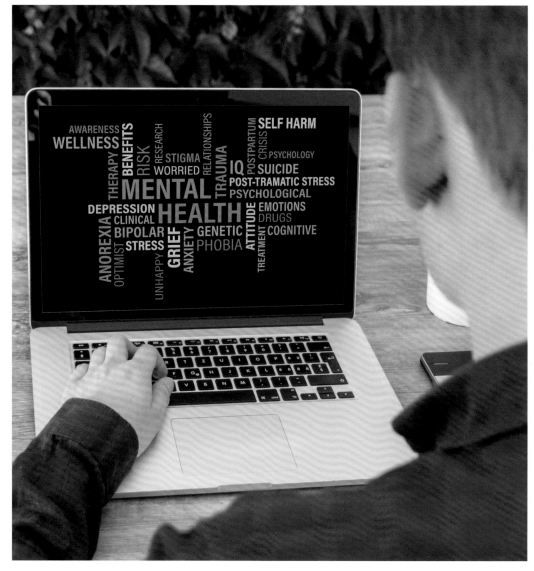

1 in 10 children have no one to talk to in school when they are worried or sad

More than one in ten children (11%) aged between 10 and 15 say they have no one to talk to or wouldn't talk to anyone in school if they feel worried or sad, according to a new survey commissioned by the Mental Health Foundation.

The survey marks the launch of our new 'Make it Count' campaign to ensure every child in the UK receives an education with mental health at its heart.

The YouGov survey of 1,323 schoolchildren in Britain also determined how feelings of being 'worried or sad' affected their wellbeing and behaviour, finding that:

> nearly four in ten
– 38% –
said that it caused them
difficulty with going to sleep

> more than a quarter
– 27% –
said they got into
fights or arguments

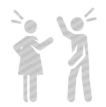

> more than one in four
– 26% –
said that it caused them to
struggle to do their homework

> more than one in four
– 27% –
didn't want to be
around others

The campaign is being launched at a time when there is already widespread evidence of a mental health crisis among young people. According to Public Health England, 10% of children and young people in England (aged five to 16) have a clinically diagnosable mental health problem.

Dr Antonis Kousoulis, Associate Director at the Mental Health Foundation:

'Our survey provides shocking further evidence of the growing crisis in the mental health of children. Nearly half a million children** in the country have no one to speak to at school when they are experiencing feelings of sadness or worry. That is plainly unacceptable.

'We believe that many mental health problems are preventable, but for prevention to work for children, changes need to take place in our schools, from primary level upwards. This is why we are campaigning for mental health to have much greater priority in our children's education.

'We know there are many schools that are doing excellent things in this area, often in difficult circumstances, but this needs to keep improving and be consistent in all schools.

'If we are not tackling mental health problems early, then we risk failing the next generation right at the start of their lives.'

Supporting the campaign, Melinda Messenger, TV presenter and mum of three said:

'As a parent of three children, I would feel 100% safer in the knowledge that while they are at school their mental health was treated with the same importance as reading and writing. This is why I am backing the Mental Health Foundation's Make it Count campaign.

'You put a lot of trust into sending your young people out into the world and under the care of others. School should be the one place where, if something comes up that they need to speak about, there should be someone they feel they can turn to.'

Rebecca Harris is an Assistant Head and SENCO at Heathfield Infant and Wilnecote Junior Schools:

'Our staff have spent a long time researching and considering how to support our pupils' mental health and emotional wellbeing following an increase in anxiety, depression, self-harming and many other alarming symptoms in our children.

'We created a new system that develops children's resilience and teaches skills in how to handle situations they may encounter.

'While we acknowledge we still have a long way to go, supporting the mental health of our pupils underpins everything. Schools must collaborate with mental health charities and professionals who can support them in developing our future adults.

'To that end, we need governmental policy that prioritises emotional wellbeing as a foundation to learning.'

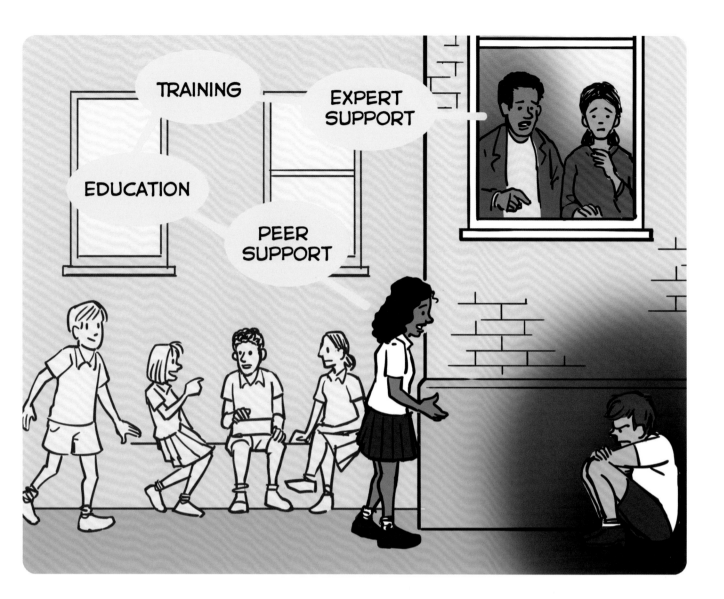

How can government and schools help 'Make it Count'?

1. Measurement

Let's help school leaders understand what works by introducing a mental wellbeing measure in schools.

2. Training

Let's give teachers the knowledge and confidence to make schools mentally healthy places by guaranteeing at least one day's training a year on learning about children's mental health.

3. Education

Let's guarantee all school children a minimum of one hour a week of the new health education curriculum focused on how to stay mentally well and seek help, delivered by well-trained teachers.

4. Peer education

Let's help young people support one another and break down the stigma often associated with mental health by introducing a peer-led mental health programme in every school.

5. Expert support

Let's provide independent counsellors in every school to help give pupils the timely support they need.

10 October 2018

All figures, unless otherwise stated, are from YouGov Plc. Total sample size was 1,359 children aged 10 to 15, of which 1,323 were in school. Fieldwork was undertaken between 14th - 26th September 2018. The survey was carried out online.

The figures have been weighted and are representative of all GB children (aged 10-15).

*When asked 'Which of the following people at your school would you talk to if you felt worried or sad?' 11% said 'I don't have anyone to talk to/ wouldn't talk to anyone at school.'

** Calculations by Mental Health Foundation, using survey results and ONS population figures. ONS estimates there are 4,292,784 10 to 15 year olds in Britain.

Of these 97.28% are in school (4,176,020). Of these, 11.4% said they don't have anyone to talk to/wouldn't talk to anyone at school if they felt worried or sad. This equated to 476,066 children aged 10 to 15.

Risk and protective factors

An excerpt from the Department for Education's advice on Mental Health and Behaviour in Schools.

Factors that put children at risk

Certain individuals and groups are more at risk of developing mental health problems than others. These risks can relate to the child themselves, to their family, or to their community or life events. These risk factors are listed in the table below.

Risk factors are cumulative. For example, children exposed to multiple risks such as social disadvantage, family adversity and cognitive or attention problems are much more likely to develop behavioural problems. Longitudinal analysis of data for 16,000 children suggested that boys with five or more risk factors were almost 11 times more likely to develop conduct disorder under the age of ten than boys with no risk factors. Girls of a similar age with five or more risk factors were 19 times more likely to develop the disorder than those with no risk factors.

Factors that make children more resilient

Research suggests that there is a complex interplay between the risk factors in children's lives, and the protective factors which can promote their resilience. As social disadvantage and the number of stressful life events accumulate for children, more protective factors are needed to act as a counterbalance. The key protective factors which build resilience to mental health problems are shown alongside the risk factors in the table, below.

In order to promote positive mental health, it is important that schools have an understanding of the protective factors that can enable pupils to be resilient when they encounter problems and challenges. The role that schools play in promoting the resilience of their pupils is particularly important for children with less supportive home lives, who may not have a trusted adult they can talk to. Schools should be a safe and affirming place for children where they can develop a sense of belonging and feel able to trust and talk openly with adults about their problems.

Risk and protective factors that are believed to be associated with mental health outcomes

	Risk factors	Protective factors
In the child	⇨ Genetic influences ⇨ Low IQ and learning disabilities ⇨ Specific development delay or neurodiversity ⇨ Communication difficulties ⇨ Difficult temperament ⇨ Physical illness ⇨ Academic failure ⇨ Low self-esteem	⇨ Outgoing temperament as an infant ⇨ Good communication skills, sociability ⇨ Being a planner and having a belief in control ⇨ Humour ⇨ A positive attitude ⇨ Experiences of success and achievement ⇨ Faith or spirituality ⇨ Capacity to reflect
In the family	⇨ Overt parental conflict including domestic violence ⇨ Family breakdown (including where children are taken into care or adopted) ⇨ Inconsistent or unclear discipline ⇨ Hostile and rejecting relationships ⇨ Failure to adapt to a child's changing needs	

	Risk factors	Protective factors
	⇨ Physical, sexual, emotional abuse, or neglect ⇨ Parental psychiatric illness ⇨ Parental criminality, alcoholism or personality disorder ⇨ Death and loss – including loss of friendship	⇨ At least one good parent-child relationship (or one supportive adult) ⇨ Affection ⇨ Clear, consistent discipline ⇨ Support for education ⇨ Supportive long-term relationship or the absence of severe discord
In the school	⇨ Bullying including online (cyber) ⇨ Discrimination ⇨ Breakdown in or lack of positive friendships ⇨ Deviant peer influences ⇨ Peer pressure ⇨ Peer on peer abuse ⇨ Poor pupil to teacher/school staff relationships	⇨ Clear policies on behaviour and bullying ⇨ Staff behaviour policy (also known as code of conduct) ⇨ 'Open door' policy for children to raise problems ⇨ A whole-school approach to promoting good mental health ⇨ Good pupil to teacher/school staff relationships ⇨ Positive classroom management ⇨ A sense of belonging ⇨ Positive peer influences ⇨ Positive friendships ⇨ Effective safeguarding and child protection policies. ⇨ An effective early help process ⇨ Understand their role in and be part of effective multi-agency working ⇨ Appropriate procedures to ensure staff are confident to/can raise concerns about policies and processes, and know they will be dealt with fairly and effectively
In the community	⇨ Socio-economic disadvantage ⇨ Homelessness ⇨ Disaster, accidents, war or other overwhelming events ⇨ Discrimination ⇨ Exploitation, including by criminal gangs and organised crime groups, trafficking, online abuse, sexual exploitation and the influences of extremism leading to radicalisation ⇨ Other significant life events	⇨ Wider supportive network ⇨ Good housing ⇨ High standard of living ⇨ High morale school with positive policies for behaviour, attitudes and anti-bullying ⇨ Opportunities for valued social roles ⇨ Range of sport/leisure activities

The above information is reprinted with kind permission from Gov.uk © Crown copyright 2019

www.gov.co.uk

Funding for mental health services fails to reach the frontline

By Keith Cooper

Mental health services for children and young people are still 'poorly funded' despite significant Government investment in services, frontline staff believe.

This is the warning from nine out of ten health professionals surveyed for a new BMA paper, which examines the financial state of mental health services, including perinatal and psychological therapy services.

Analysis of data from official sources and Freedom of Information (FoI) requests found evidence that the recent, and welcome, hike in central funding was failing to reach the frontline.

Despite the increase, many clinical commissioning groups CCGs, which buy and plan care, were either maintaining or reducing cash flows to mental health trusts – as they in turn struggled to cope with rising demand.

'Despite some geographic variations,' the paper states, 'there appears to be no obvious uplift in spending in recent years.'

It adds: 'Insufficient funding is one of the most significant barriers that limits doctors' ability to provide optimal mental healthcare to patients.'

Figures in the report point to a 9.1% increase in the prevalence of depression between 2015–16 and 2016–17 and a 44 per cent increase in contacts with mental health and learning disability services between 2014–15 and 2016–17.

FoI requests by the BMA for the report indicate the CCGs have also prioritised talking therapies for people with relatively mild mental health conditions over those with more severe ones.

Waiting to talk

Eight out of ten CCGs said they spent more on increasing access to psychological therapies than talking therapies suitable for patients in secondary care, under the care of a psychiatrist. This finding supports those of the BMA's recently published investigation which revealed waiting times of up to two years for secondary care talking therapies and that most trusts and CCGs do not keep track of them.

The 'de-prioritisation' of psychological therapies in secondary care was concerning, the funding paper states, as official figures show a 63 per cent increase in demand for such care between 2012-13 and 2016-17.

The report recommends a funding increase across the NHS and an expansion of the data set for mental health to cover perinatal mental health and psychological therapies.

BMA consultants committee deputy chair and child and adolescent psychiatrist Gary Wannan said: 'These findings

are further evidence that funding for mental health services are failing to get through to the frontline at a time of escalating demand.

'Given the multiple pressures on commissioners across all parts of the NHS, this is not surprising. We have just experienced the worst winter ever in the NHS; the pressures from the acute sector shows no sign of letting up anytime soon.

'It's also of concern that there remain huge gaps in the official data on mental health funding. How can we know how far we're along the road to parity of esteem without the data to guide us?'

19 February 2018

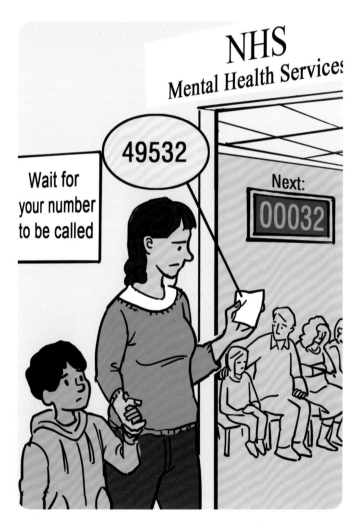

Mental health: there are fewer beds, nurses and psychiatry trainees than in 2010

By Grace Rahman

In brief

Claim

The number of hospital beds for people with acute mental health conditions has fallen by 30%.

Conclusion

These years aren't comparable due to a change in collection method from 2010. Between 2010 and 2017 there was a 22% drop.

"The number of hospital beds for people with acute mental health conditions, where a consultant psychiatrist is on hand to oversee treatment, has fallen by almost 30% since 2009."

The Observer, 21 July 2018

The number of overnight beds for those suffering with mental health issues, mental health nurses and psychiatrists in training in the NHS in England have all dropped since 2009.

Mental health beds

Using comparable figures since 2010, the average number of mental illness beds per year has dropped by 22% from 23,400 to 18,300.

The 30% drop claim compares years before and after a change in the way the data was collected in 2010, which means fewer bed types are now counted. The figure used in *The Observer* compares 2009/10 with 2017/18, which are not comparable.

NHS England said that since 2013/14, the drop may have been affected by trusts reclassifying beds so they are no longer 'consultant-led', and are instead run by 'multidisciplinary teams'.

This is for beds under the care of consultants, so won't cover all beds for people suffering with a mental illness.

The number of hospital beds in general has fallen over the last 30 years, despite rising population and patient numbers, mainly because of advances in medicine.

The number of mental illness overnight beds dropped by 62% in the 20 years to 2009. The King's Fund put this decrease down to the 'policy shift to providing care for people with mental health problems and learning disabilities in the community rather than in institutional settings'.

Mental health nurses

The number of full-time equivalent (FTE) mental health and learning disabilities nurses dropped by 16%, or by around 7,500 between September 2009 and September 2010.

The figures quoted in the claim compared the number of mental health and learning disability nurses between September 2009 and March 2018, but as the number of nurses working in the NHS in England changes throughout the year this isn't a fair comparison.

The majority of these nurses (90% in March 2018) are mental health nurses, with the rest working with patients with learning disabilities.

10% of these nurses work with people with learning disabilities and difficulties, and are included in the number of mental health nurses because of a wider definition of 'mental health nurses' used by NHS Digital, which publishes the figures.

Just looking at nurses working in mental health, the number has fallen by 13%, or by 5,200 between September 2009 and September 2017.

Trainee psychiatrists

Following their two foundation years of training after medical school, junior doctors can choose to specialise.

There were the equivalent of around 3,200 full-time junior doctors specialising in psychiatry training in September 2009. That number had fallen by around 500, or 15% by September 2017 – the most recent comparable figures.

There were around 2,600 FTE junior doctors in psychiatry training in March 2018.

A report from Health Education England published in 2017 said not enough newly qualified doctors were 'choosing/able to train in psychiatry' and that there was a higher proportion of unfilled core psychiatry training posts than in any other speciality.

It said that there were 'low direct transition rates' from core psychiatry training into more specialised training and that the field relied on non-UK doctors choosing to specialise. It also said the workforce heavily relied on doctors who are neither training nor consultants, for which there isn't 'a secure supply pipeline'.

26 July 2018

These black women felt excluded by mainstream mental health charities – so they started their own

By Victoria Sanusi

Two young black women in London found themselves feeling so excluded from mainstream mental health charities that they decided to create one, while dealing with mental health problems of their own.

According to the Mental Health Foundation, black and minority ethnic groups living in the UK are more likely to be diagnosed with mental health problems and more likely to experience a poor outcome from treatment.

Young black people aren't being engaged

'Nowadays, diversity seems to be at the top of everyone's agenda and I think mainstream charities are trying to take this on board, which you can see through their ads and campaigns,' Vanessa Boachie, founder of Inside Out UK told *i*.

'However, the research tells us that black British people are most affected by mental health issues in the UK and when you look at the people who are in charge of these charities and designing the programmes and campaigns, most of the time they are not black British.'

'So can you really empathise and create the right support if you don't understand the struggle? Is that why black British young people may not be as engaged?'

In April 2017, a then 21-year-old Boachie created her own charity, Inside Out UK, to provide preventative strategies to reduce the risk of young black people developing severe mental health problems and to promote positive mental health.

Lack of services

While working in a rehabilitation recovery home to gain clinical experience to become a clinical psychologist, she said what she found shocking was the lack of services available, due to the reduction of government funding and the services that were available were either oversubscribed or not appealing for young people to want to learn more.

'I worked with clients who were diagnosed with schizophrenia and associated mental health disorders such as depression, bipolar disorder, anxiety disorder and OCD,' she said.

Her experience there really opened her eyes to what people with severe mental health issues deal with, and she was curious as to what could have been done to prevent them from being in that position.

Similar to Boachie, 23-year-old Saida Odutayo feels mainstream charities aren't inclusive. 'The sad thing is mainstream mental health organisations are just not representative of African and Caribbean people as well as Asian people," she told *i*.

Odutayo became the founder of SAIE in August 2017 and registered the charity a few months later.

Her dissertation focused on the mental health of black girls and investigated how social stigmas and parental attitudes were stopping them from accessing mental health services, inspiring her to start the charity.

Odutayo said the interviews she conducted were horrific.

'One person I interviewed had a father who was a psychiatrist, who prescribed medication to his patients but to his daughter he consistently

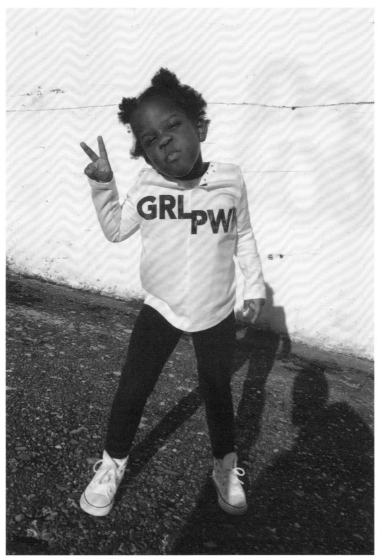

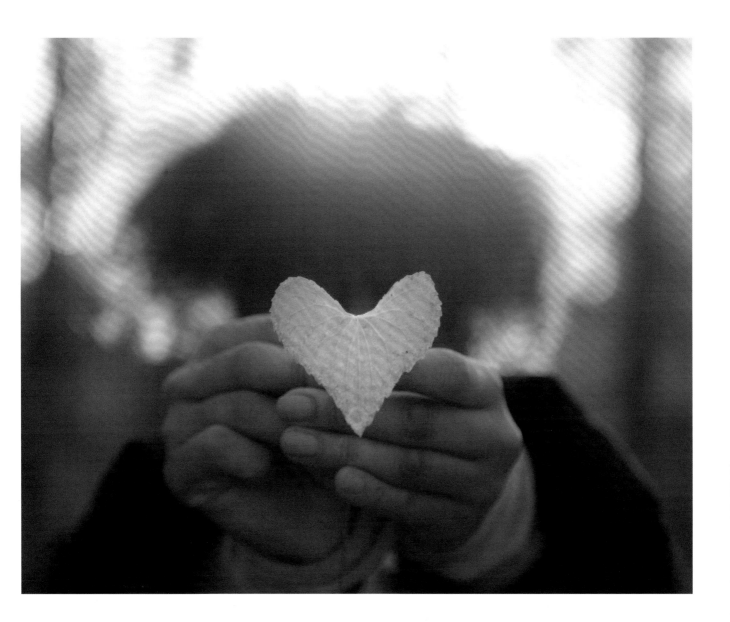

told her that her mental health issues are a result of her non-existent relationship with God," Odutayo said to *i*.

'Another had attempted to commit suicide on three occasions and when her mother found her said she would bring shame to the family if she was to die like that.'

Now she feels compelled to do more to oppose the neglected, on-going issue in minority communities, where mental health is heavily stigmatised or ignored. Odutayo herself is dealing with depression while she runs the charity and works as a prison officer.

Events involve people in conversations about mental health

Both Boachie and Odutayo's charities put on events with people from the black community, encouraging people to come down and talk about mental health. For some attendees it's the first time they've had this sort of conversation in public.

A total of 500 people have attended Boachie's events. When asked how it made her feel that black people are so engaged with her charity, she said: 'It's not really about how I feel, I just want people to be aware and educated about mental health so they can have the knowledge and skills to equip themselves and others when challenging situations arise.

'It means the information we provide is coming from someone they can relate to and if that increases the impact, then I guess I'm closer to fulfilling my purpose on this earth.' As for Odutayo, she said it feels great knowing that black women come to her organisation for help and champion what they do as a charity. 'Since the launch, we knew black women would come through and be at the forefront speaking up about some of the challenges they face. Its even representative within our team of volunteers,' she added.

Now her focus is maintaining the relationship she has with black women but do more to reach out to black men, who she said do not speak out enough.

15 May 2018

An interest rate rise may put thousands at risk of mental health problems

An article from The Conversation.

By Christopher Boyce

THE CONVERSATION

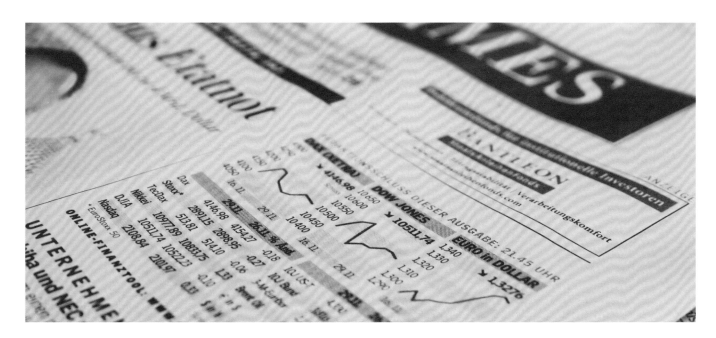

After nine years of interest rates below one per cent, it seems the Bank of England will announce a rise before long. As pay growth picks up and inflation hits its two per cent target, a rate rise would – it is argued – ward off potential risks of inflation in the medium term.

But another factor to bear in mind is that a rate rise could also have serious repercussions for people's mental health. A large portion of the population have high, possibly unsustainable, levels of debt and a higher interest rate is likely to increase the burden of repaying some of that debt. It will, therefore, likely increase their levels of mental distress.

In recent research that colleagues and I published in the *Journal of Affective Disorders*, we explored how Bank of England interest rate changes from 1995 to 2008 influenced people's mental health. What we found is that for each one per cent increase in interest rates, there was a 2.6 per cent increase in the incidence of mental health issues experienced by those heavily indebted.

Although there is always some margin for error in statistical estimates, this would translate to 20,000 additional cases of mental health difficulty in the UK. As well as the obvious health cost here, there is also a financial cost. Since one case of mental health has been estimated to cost somewhere in the order of £8,000, in terms of absences from work and lost quality of life, this would have an overall cost to society of £156 million.

Although over-indebtedness is well known to be bad for people's mental health, our study is the first to show that there is a direct relationship between central bank interest rate decisions and mental health. This raises the question of whether central banks should also consider how their decisions influence population mental health.

Wellbeing-based policy

There has been a growing interest in using non-economic indicators to guide public policy, with the suggestion that more emphasis perhaps ought to be placed on psychological outcomes. Some economic objectives, such as economic growth and inflation, are often not strongly linked to changes in mental health and wellbeing.

With regard to monetary policy, some have argued that since unemployment is considerably worse for mental health than inflation, greater emphasis should be placed on reducing unemployment than maintaining price stability. Plus, income growth has limited effects on general wellbeing when compared with other factors, such as health, relationships and personality, and it has been shown that the avoidance of income losses matters much more for wellbeing than the pursuit of income gains.

But the Bank of England's objective is purely economic. Namely 'to maintain price stability', as defined by the Government's two per cent inflation target. And, subject to that, to support the Government's economic policies, including those for growth and employment. It is generally agreed that ensuring price stability is the best way that central banks can support long-term economic growth, as it fosters greater confidence in the economy and encourages investment.

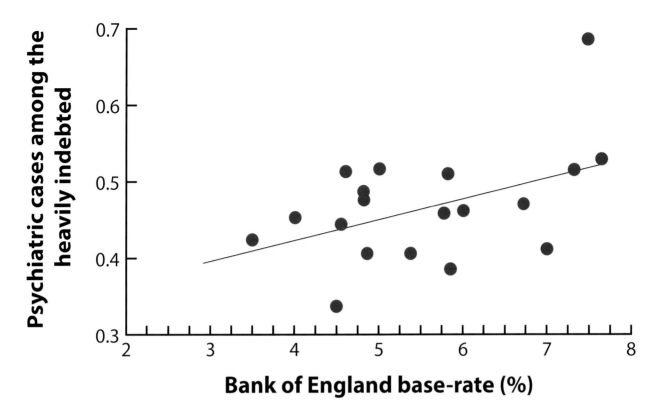

The link between interest rate changes and mental health. Boyce et al. (2018), CC BY-ND

Price stability is generally maintained by ensuring that the money supply increases at the same rate as economic growth or output. If money supply increases faster than output, then it is believed that this will result in inflation. A central bank may increase money supply at a faster rate than real output, to inject more demand into an economy. This can generate higher economic growth and lower the rate of unemployment, which can be helpful during times of recession.

Of course, a decision not to increase rates may cost the economy much more than the loss from increased mental health cases of the £156 million estimated earlier. An increase in inflation expectations may in the longer term, for example, lower overall economic confidence and discourage investment. Plus, having low interest rates for too long may encourage people to take on levels of debt that become unsustainable when rates are higher. Rates that were too low for too long to obtain economic objectives may themselves have been a contributor to the present state of indebtedness.

Don't ignore the repercussions

The central bank's objectives do not necessarily need to change to anything but economic ones. But our research does clearly illustrate that the pursuit of economic objectives will likely have painful repercussions for individuals. These should be acknowledged, forewarned and where possible, countered.

For example, this may take the form of helping people avert excessive indebtedness, strong public health warnings around indebtedness levels, and ensuring adequate mental health support for those that have become heavily indebted.

There is also an alternative approach to conducting monetary policy that may meet economic objectives, yet still help protect people's mental health. Over the last decade, central banks tried to maintain price stability by injecting trillions into financial markets by buying up bonds and assets so as to increase the money supply.

This quantitative easing approach has been criticised because it had very little impact on the economy since it didn't give regular people more money in their pocket to spend. Giving money directly to individuals might have been more effective. It would likely also have helped decrease people's debt burden, and therefore the pressures on mental health. Mental health issues are often more debilitating than many physical health issues, yet the available resources to help those in psychological difficulty remain vastly insufficient. Not only do we need comprehensive strategies for helping people cope with psychological difficulties directly, but it is important to recognise that mental health links to the economy. We must therefore create an economic environment that is supportive to people's mental health.

Christopher Boyce is a research fellow at the behavioural science centre at the University of Stirling.

10 May 2018

Five lifestyle changes to enhance your mood and mental health

An article from The Conversation.

THE CONVERSATION

When someone is diagnosed with a mental health disorder such as depression or anxiety, first line treatments usually include psychological therapies and medication. What's not always discussed are the changeable lifestyle factors that influence our mental health.

Even those who don't have a mental health condition may still be looking for ways to further improve their mood, reduce stress, and manage their day-to-day mental health.

It can be empowering to make positive life changes. While time restrictions and financial limitations may affect some people's ability to make such changes, we all have the ability to make small meaningful changes.

Here are five lifestyle changes to get you started:

1. Improve your diet and start moving

Wholefoods such as leafy green vegetables, legumes, wholegrains, lean red meat and seafood, provide nutrients that are important for optimal brain function. These foods contain magnesium, folate, zinc and essential fatty acids.

Foods rich in polyphenols, such as berries, tea, dark chocolate, wine and certain herbs, also play an important role in brain function.

In terms of exercise, many types of fitness activities are potentially beneficial – from swimming, to jogging, to lifting weights, or playing sports . Even just getting the body moving by taking a brisk walk or doing active housework is a positive step.

Activities which also involve social interaction and exposure to nature can potentially increase mental well-being even further .

General exercise guidelines recommend getting at least 30 minutes of moderate activity on most days during the week (about 150 minutes total over the week). But even short bouts of activity can provide an immediate elevation of mood.

2. Reduce your vices

Managing problem-drinking or substance misuse is an obvious health recommendation. People with alcohol and drug problems have a greater likelihood than average of having a mental illness, and have far poorer health outcomes.

Some research has shown that a little alcohol consumption (in particular wine) may have beneficial effects on preventing depression. Other recent data, however, has revealed that light alcohol consumption does not provide any beneficial effects on brain function.

Stopping smoking is also an important step, as nicotine-addicted people are constantly at the mercy of a withdrawal-craving cycle, which profoundly affects mood. It may take time to address the initial symptoms of stopping nicotine, but the brain chemistry will adapt in time.

Quitting smoking is associated with better mood and reduced anxiety.

3. Prioritise rest and sleep

Sleep hygiene techniques aim to improve sleep quality and help treat insomnia. They include adjusting caffeine use, limiting exposure to the bed (regulating your sleep time and

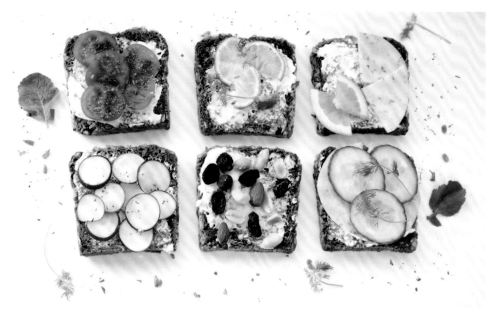

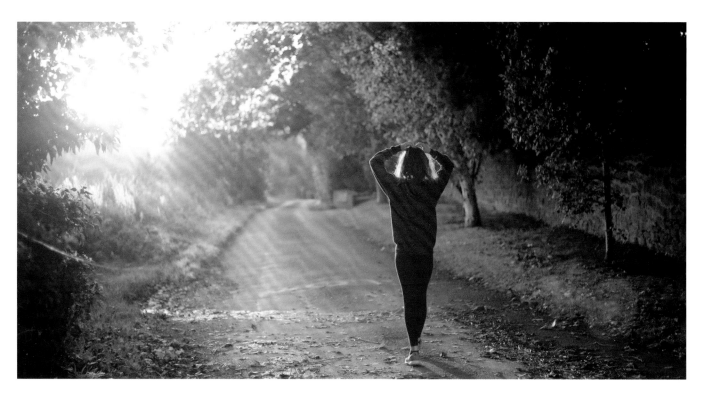

having a limited time to sleep), and making sure you get up at a similar time in the morning.

Some people are genetically wired towards being more of a morning or evening person, so we need to ideally have some flexibility in this regard (especially with work schedules).

It's also important not to force sleep – if you can't get to sleep within around 20 minutes, it may be best to get up and focus the mind on an activity (with minimal light and stimulation) until you feel tired.

The other mainstay of better sleep is to reduce exposure to light – especially blue light from laptops and smartphones – prior to sleep. This will increase the secretion of melatonin, which helps you get to sleep.

Getting enough time for relaxation and leisure activities is important for regulating stress. Hobbies can also enhance mental health, particularly if they involve physical activity.

4. Get a dose of nature

When the sun is shining, many of us seem to feel happier. Adequate exposure to sunshine helps levels of the mood-maintaining chemical serotonin. It also boosts vitamin D levels, which also has an effect on mental health, and helps at the appropriate time to regulate our sleep-wake cycle.

The benefits of sun exposure need to be balanced with the risk of skin cancer, so take into account the recommendations for sun exposure based on the time of day/year and your skin colour.

You might also consider limiting your exposure to environmental toxins, chemicals and pollutants, including 'noise' pollution, and cutting down on your mobile phone, computer and TV use if they're excessive.

An antidote to this can be simply spending time in nature. Studies show time in the wilderness can improve self-esteem and mood. In some parts of Asia, spending time in a forest (known as forest bathing) is considered a mental health prescription.

A natural extension of spending time in flora is also the positive effect that animals have on us. Research suggests having a pet has many positive effects, and animal-assisted therapy (with horses, cats, dogs and even dolphins) may also boost feelings of well-being.

5. Reach out when you need help

Positive lifestyle changes aren't a replacement for medication or psychological therapy but, rather, as something people can undertake themselves on top of their treatment.

While many lifestyle changes can be positive, some changes (such as avoiding junk foods, alcohol or giving up smoking) may be challenging if being used as a psychological crutch. They might need to be handled delicately, and with professional support.

Strict advice promoting abstinence, or a demanding diet or exercise regime, may cause added suffering, potentially provoking guilt if you can't meet these expectations. So go easy on yourself.

That said, take a moment to reflect how you feel mentally after a nutritious wholefood meal, a good night's sleep (free of alcohol) or a walk in nature with a friend.

9 October 2018

For the first time, print media reporting of mental health is significantly more balanced and responsible with more coverage than ever before – latest study shows

But worryingly, the reporting of violence and mental illness, and schizophrenia continues to be stigmatising.

The 2016 figures have been released by Time to Change as part of 'Mind Over Matter', its ongoing collaboration with the Institute of Psychiatry, Psychology & Neuroscience, King's College London, which examines the reporting of mental illness in the UK print media.

For the first time since the study started in 2008 there were significantly more anti-stigmatising articles (50%) than stigmatising (35%) articles. The remainder of articles were mixed (6%) or neutral (9%).

Stigmatising refers to articles which portray people with mental health problems as a danger to others, or a hopeless victim, as behaving strangely, or being a problem for others. Whereas, articles were rated as anti-stigmatising if they offered a more sympathetic portrayal, or focused on recovery and treatment or promoted mental health. The study was based on an analysis of articles on mental illness from 27 local and national UK newspapers, on two randomly selected days of each month during 2016.

The results for 2016 have been published to coincide with this year's Virgin Money Giving Mind Media Awards. Other findings include:

2016 had the highest number of articles covering issues related to mental health since the study began (1,738 articles compared with 941 in 2014, the highest previous sample size), showing how mainstream the topic has now become.

The most common sources for articles were people with mental health problems, both public figures and general public, reflecting the increasing numbers speaking out about the issue

But the most frequent stigmatising elements in reporting were 'danger to others' and 'hopeless victim', demonstrating there is still more work to be done to challenge outdated stereotypes.

And, worryingly, reporting on schizophrenia was more often stigmatising than anti-stigmatising, the only mental illness diagnosis to see this.

Time to Change is run by mental health charities Mind and Rethink Mental Illness. Its director, Sue Baker said: 'The media can be incredibly powerful when it comes to educating and influencing the public about mental health. When done well, the media helps to raise awareness, challenge attitudes and dispel myths. But sensationalist journalism can overplay the risk of violence, promote fear and mistrust and widen the gap of understanding.

'The findings from this latest study shows we're heading in the right direction but there's more still to be done, particularly when it comes to challenging misconceptions around mental illness and violence.'

Benjamin Damtten, 43, has experienced first hand the impact of sensationalist media coverage; he said 'A lot of people who hear the word schizophrenia are scared. They are scared because all they have to go on is what they see on the news, which is the "madman" with a machete. I am the opposite of that. I sit on my own in my house, sometimes crying, because I am terrified. I am scared to face the world.'

'I also think people in my area know I have schizophrenia and they treat me differently. They pull their children away from me or they move away at the bus stop. I think "What do they think I'm going to do? Do they think I'm violent?"'

17 November 2017

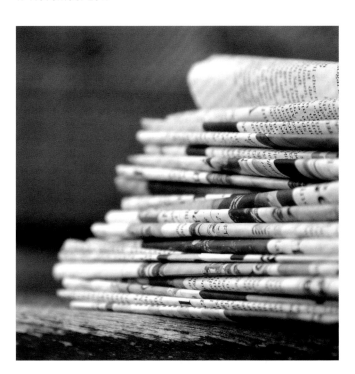

Gaming addiction can be treated on the NHS after it is declared a medical disorder

By Charles Hymas

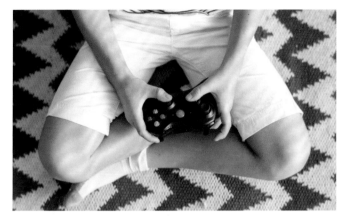

Children hooked on addictive video games like *Fortnite* will be able to seek treatment on the NHS after video gaming is classified as a medical disorder by the World Health Organization (WHO) next week.

The WHO will on Monday notify governments around the world that they will be expected to incorporate 'gaming disorder' into their health systems.

The move comes amid increasing evidence of young players suffering psychological distress and family breakdown as a result of their addiction.

This week *The Daily Telegraph* revealed one 15-year-old gaming addict in London had been hospitalised for eight weeks and off school for a year after losing the confidence to go outside.

The disorder will be added to the WHO's International Classification of Disease which means that those diagnosed will be entitled to be treated by the NHS.

The guidelines state that for a diagnosis a victim's behaviour must be 'of sufficient severity to result in significant impairment in personal, family, social, educational, occupational or other important areas of functioning.' They would also normally be expected to have suffered it for at least a year.

Dr Vladimir Poznyak, of the WHO's Mental Health and Substance Abuse department, told *The Daily Telegraph* that studies suggested between 1% and 6% of adolescents and young people may be afflicted by gaming addiction although these were not as yet diagnosed victims.

He also revealed the WHO considered social media addiction as part of its four-year investigation into the impact on health of excessive use of the internet, computers and smart phones. It had been decided there was not currently sufficient evidence to justify its classification as a disorder.

This week *The Daily Telegraph* launched its 'Duty of Care' campaign, calling on the Government to make social media and online gaming companies subject to a statutory duty to protect children from harms such as addiction, bullying and grooming.

The classification of gaming disorder was welcomed yesterday by the Royal College of Psychiatrists. Dr Henrietta Bowden-Jones, the college's expert on behavioural addiction, said it was an important recognition of the plight of an 'extremely vulnerable' group of largely young people.

'There's no NHS services to provide support for them,' she said. 'I strongly believe we should make available across the country services annexed to our existing addiction units that can be commissioned to provide help, advice and behaviour modification to this group.

'These are not people who have been drinking for years. These are young new cases where their compulsive behaviour is impacting negatively on their home, family and usually their schoolwork.'

She said it could also entail proper screening and data collection to establish the scale of addiction: 'I have calls every day from people wanting to discuss their children and [the video game] *Fortnite*, and their children and gaming.'

Mark Griffiths, Professor of Behavioural Addiction at Nottingham Trent University and a member of the WHO working group, said it was vindication of his 30 year, work in addiction but doubted the NHS would be able to devote the necessary resources to treatment. He added: 'It's no different to gambling or other addictions.'

Earlier this week Professor Griffiths revealed in *The Daily Telegraph* that high-quality studies showed 4% of adolescents could be classed as at risk of internet addiction, equivalent to one child in every secondary class in the country.

Dr Richard Graham, a leading adolescent consultant psychiatrist, called for the NHS to fund a specialist centre to treat patients suffering from technology addiction.

The demand for such a centre, which would follow a similar model to the NHS's offering for gambling addicts, who are treated by the National Problem Gambling Clinic, is 'substantial', said Dr Graham.

'The centre should maybe have a residential aspect for people who really can't manage,' he said.

'We are going to be living with devices around us, on and and in us for the foreseeable future so the formation of this centre can't wait.'

15 June 2018

LSD and magic mushrooms could heal damaged brain cells in people suffering from depression, study shows

Psychedelics could be 'next generation' of safer treatments for mental health.

By Alex Matthews-King

Psychedelic drugs like LSD and ecstasy ingredient MDMA have been shown to stimulate the growth of new branches and connections between brain cells which could help address conditions like depression and addiction.

Researchers in California have demonstrated these substances, banned as illicit drugs in many countries, are capable of rewiring parts of the brain in a way that lasts well beyond the drugs' effects.

This means psychedelics could be the 'next generation' of treatments for mental health disorders which could be more effective and safer than existing options, say the study's authors from the University of California.

In previous studies by the same team, a single dose of DMT, the key ingredient in ayahuasca medicinal brews of Amazonian tribes, has been shown to help rats overcome a fear of electric shock meant to emulate post-traumatic stress disorder (PTSD).

Now they have shown this dose increases the number of branch-like dendrites sprouting from nerve cells in the rat's brain. These dendrites end at synapses where their electrical impulses are passed on to other nerve cells and underpin all brain activity. But they can atrophy and draw back in people with mental health conditions.

'One of the hallmarks of depression is that the neurites in the prefrontal cortex – a key brain region that regulates emotion, mood, and anxiety – those neurites tend to shrivel up,' says Dr David Olson, who led the research team.

These brain changes also appear in cases of anxiety, addiction and post-traumatic stress disorder and stimulating them to reconnect could help to address this.

The research, published in the journal *Cell Reports* today, looked at drugs in several classes including tryptamines, DMT and magic mushrooms; amphetamines, including MDMA; and ergolines, like LSD.

In tests on human brain cells in the lab, flies and rats, it found these substances consistently boosted brain connections.

Dr Olson compared the effects to ketamine, another illicit drug which represents one of the most important new treatments for depression in a generation, and found many psychedelics have equal or greater effects.

A ketamine nasal spray is being fast-tracked through clinical trials after it was shown to rapidly relieve major depression and suicidal thoughts in people who cannot be helped by other treatments.

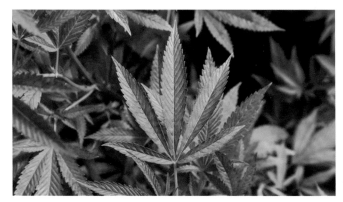

However, its use has to be weighed against its potential for abuse, and its ability to cause a form of drug-induced psychosis.

'The rapid effects of ketamine on mood and plasticity are truly astounding,' said Dr Olson. 'The big question we were trying to answer was whether or not other compounds are capable of doing what ketamine does.

'People have long assumed that psychedelics are capable of altering neuronal structure, but this is the first study that clearly and unambiguously supports that hypothesis.'

The fact that many of these drugs seem to mimic the groundbreaking benefits of ketamine opens up an array of new treatment options, which may be less open to abuse, if these drugs can make it to clinical trials.

Dr Olson said: 'Ketamine is no longer our only option. Our work demonstrates that there are a number of distinct chemical scaffolds capable of promoting plasticity like ketamine, providing additional opportunities for medicinal chemists to develop safer and more effective alternatives.'

The news that yet more banned substances could help tackle serious and debilitating disease comes as the UK Home Office is embroiled in a row over medicinal cannabis in treating epilepsy.

After months seizure-free, 12-year-old Billy Caldwell had a seizure last night after airport customs officials confiscated his prescription from Canada.

Billy had previously had the UK's only NHS medical cannabis prescription, for an oil which banished seizures that used to strike 100 times a day, but the Home Office intervened to block his GP from prescribing it.

12 June 2018

Why we invest in mental health

Everyone has mental health – and evidence shows that the benefits of physical activity on our wellbeing are profound.

Mental wellbeing is a key objective in our strategy, Towards an Active Nation. The benefits of sport and physical activity on our mental health are endless: improved mood, decreased chance of depression and anxiety, and a better and more balanced lifestyle.

The Government's Sporting Future strategy has mental wellbeing at its heart. And we're already investing in projects across the country – from small community programmes to regional and national pilots.

So far we've invested £8,160,436 of government and National Lottery funding.

Doing sport isn't just about playing in a team or joining a club.

Any kind of physical activity can boost mental wellbeing – from swimming to walking and yoga to dance.

How physical activity helps mental health

There are various ways that physical activity helps mental health, including:

Improved mood – Studies show that physical activity has a positive impact on our mood. One study asked people to rate their mood after a period of exercise (i.e. walking or gardening) and after inactivity (i.e. reading a book). Researchers found that people felt more awake, calmer and more content after physical activity.

Reduced stress – Being regularly active is shown to have a beneficial impact on alleviating stress. It can help manage stressful lifestyles and can help us make better decisions when under pressure. Research on working adults shows that active people tend to have lower stress rates compared to those who are less active.

Better self-esteem – Physical activity has a big impact on our self-esteem – that's how we feel about ourselves and our perceived self-worth. This is a key indicator of mental wellbeing. Those with improved self-esteem can cope better with stress and improve relationships with others.

Depression and anxiety – Exercise has been described as a 'wonder drug' in preventing and managing mental health. Many GPs now prescribe physical activity for depression, either on its own or in conjunction with other treatments. It is effective at both preventing onset of depression and in terms of managing symptoms.

July 2017

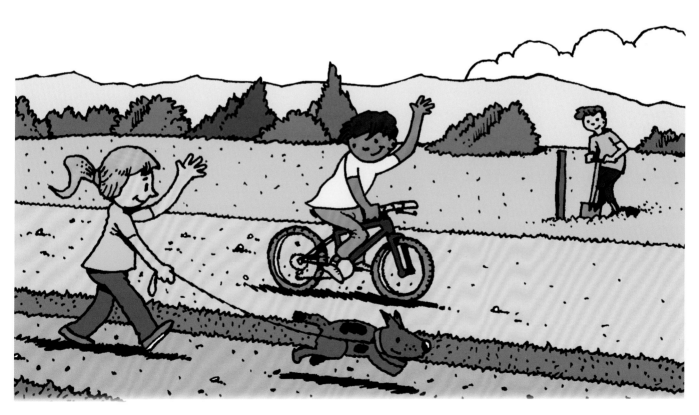

Report shows that therapy dogs may reduce risk of self-harm in prisoners

Therapy dogs can help prisoners to restore their mental health and reduce the risk of serious self-harm, according to a report published today by Centre for Mental Health.

The report

'Restoring something lost', by Graham Durcan, is an evaluation of a pilot therapy dog scheme run by Rethink Mental Illness in three prisons in the North East of England.

It finds that the therapy dogs, Magic and Cooper, had a calming influence on prisoners, helped increase coping skills and strategies, and provided a safe space for them to explore ways of expressing and processing their emotions.

The project was provided with grant funding by Her Majesty's Prison & Probation Service (HMPPS) as part of a programme to pilot, develop and test initiatives which may reduce the risk of self-harm or self-inflicted death in prison. The two therapy dogs worked with both women and men (including young men) in three prisons. They were handled by Rethink Mental Illness practitioners who were experienced in working in prisons and with people with mental health problems, and who were also experts in dog handling and agility.

Benefits of therapy dogs

Levels of self-harm rose by 20% in prisons in 2018, and at least nine out of ten prisoners has at least one mental health problem. We found clear benefits of the therapy dog scheme including a significant reduction of the severity of need (including rates of self-harm).

One of the participants in the programme: '…I can't describe it, but it takes me back to a happier place and somehow that helps me feel better about myself…'

Dr Graham Durcan, Centre for Mental Health associate director said: 'We saw positive change in the majority of the participants after their therapy dog sessions. The impact of interacting with the dogs was marked for people whose wellbeing was otherwise so poor.

'This is a stark reminder of the need to support wellbeing in prisons but also of the simple steps that could help to tackle rising levels of self-harm and to make prisons a safer and healthier environment for everyone."

Jonathan Munro, associate director for criminal justice and secure care services at Rethink Mental Illness, said: "There's a mental health crisis happening in UK prisons at the moment and we need to find creative ways to tackle it. What was unique about this project was that the team was trained in mental health, prison work and dog handling. With this specialist knowledge in all three areas we were able to really engage with prisoners, and they reported feeling a lot better as a result.'

18 December 2018

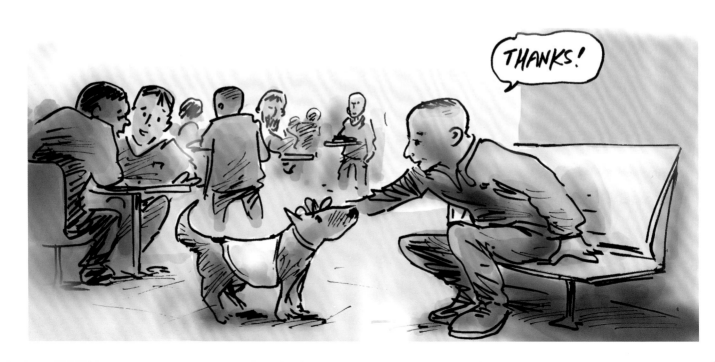

What treatments are available?

Talking treatments

Talking treatments provide a regular time and space for you to talk about your thoughts and experiences and explore difficult feelings with a trained professional. This could help you to:

- deal with a specific problem
- cope with upsetting memories or experiences
- improve your relationships
- develop more helpful ways of living day-to-day.

You may hear various terms used to describe talking treatments, including counselling, psychotherapy, therapy, talking therapy or psychological therapy. These terms are all used to describe the same general style of treatment.

There are lots of different kinds of therapy available in the UK and it's important to find a style and a therapist that you feel comfortable with.

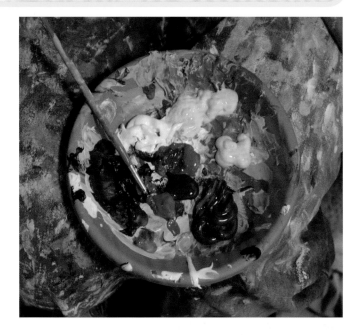

Medication

The most common type of treatment available is psychiatric medication. These drugs don't cure mental health problems, but they can ease many symptoms. Which type of drug you are offered will depend on your diagnosis. For example:

Many people find these drugs helpful, as they can lessen your symptoms and allow you to cope at work and at home. However, drugs can sometimes have unpleasant side-effects that may make you feel worse rather than better. They can also be difficult to withdraw from, or cause you physical harm if taken in too high a dose.

Arts and creative therapies

Arts and creative therapies are a way of using the arts (music, painting, dance or drama) to express and understand yourself in a therapeutic environment, with a trained therapist.

This can be especially helpful if you find it difficult to talk about your problems and how you are feeling.

Complementary and alternative therapies

Some people find complementary and alternative therapies helpful to manage stress and other common symptoms of mental health problems. These can include things like yoga, meditation, aromatherapy, hypnotherapy, herbal remedies and acupuncture.

The clinical evidence for these options is not as robust as it is for other treatments, but you may find they work for you.

October 2017 – to be revised in 2020.

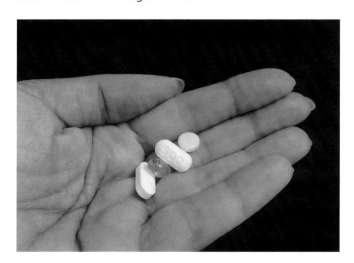

ASMR videos could be a new digital therapy for mental health

An article from **The Conversation.**

By Thomas Hostler

THE CONVERSATION

You may know 'ASMR' as the niche genre of YouTube video which people watch on tablets and laptops to help them relax, perhaps before bed or in the lull of a Sunday afternoon. These videos typically involve someone role-playing a mundane professional service, such as giving you a haircut, a massage or booking you in for a doctors' appointment.

The role-plays are usually performed in whispered voices, with the 'ASMRtist' (the term for the creators of these videos) focused on building a feeling of intimacy and emphasising any crisp sounds or slow hand movements. But what exactly is ASMR, and why do people watch these videos?

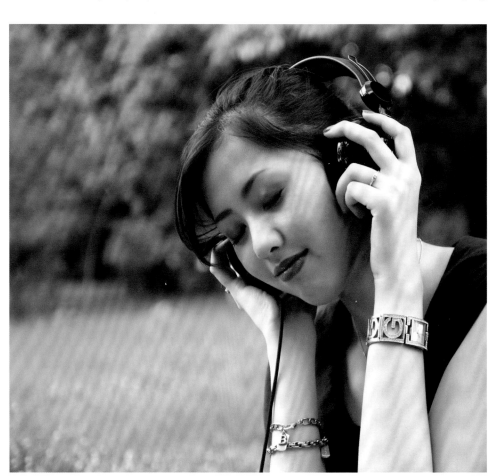

Although ASMR has been adopted as the name for these kinds of videos, it actually refers to the sensation that they are designed to induce: Autonomous Sensory Meridian Response. It is a pleasant tingling sensation that usually begins at the top of your head and spreads down your body.

If you don't experience it then it can be hard to describe, although it's not too dissimilar to goosebumps or the 'chills' you may get when listening to an epic piece of music or inspirational speech, or when gazing on an awe-inspiring scene.

It often stems from incidental triggers in everyday life. I used to experience it is as a child when having my feet measured by a shoe shop assistant. This is a good example of a scenario that contains multiple common ASMR triggers: a gentle, soft-spoken voice, precise and expert hand movements, and a sensation of being paid close attention to, but in a somewhat objectifying and professional manner. ASMR videos exaggerate and combine these triggers to attempt to induce ASMR in viewers.

It's worth noting that ASMR videos are not actually that 'niche' – some of the most popular ASMRtists have over one million subscribers, and some of their most-watched videos have over 20 million views. However, the prevalence of ASMR is difficult to estimate.

Surveys asking whether people experience ASMR disproportionally attract the attention of those who do experience it and seek out information on it. Other people may experience it but be unfamiliar with the terminology, and know it as 'brain tingles' or 'head tingles'.

The phrase 'brain orgasm' has also been used, and ASMR videos have been described as 'whisper porn', although these terms are misleading. Despite the intimate nature of ASMR videos, the sensation itself is distinctly non-sexual and is pleasurable in the same way as a blissful meditative state might be.

Many ASMR videos have more in common with instructional videos or craft-making demonstrations. Indeed, the Bob Ross painting series, *The Joy of Painting*, from the 1980s is an unintentional ASMR classic.

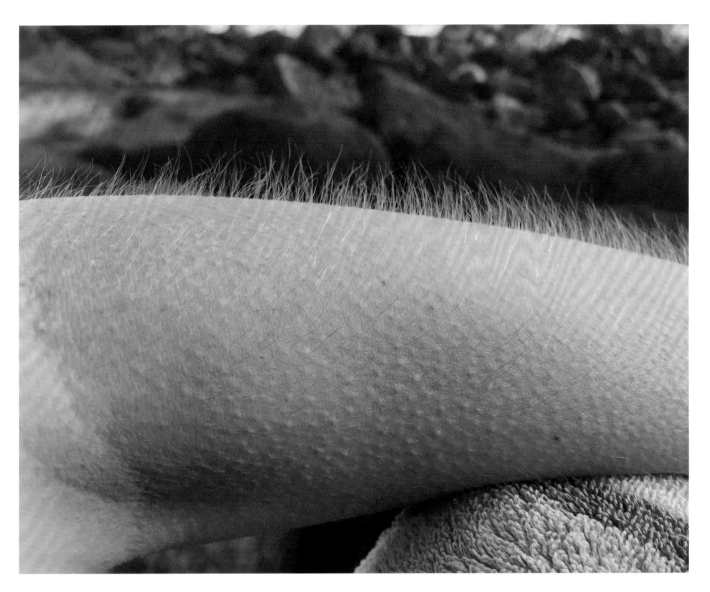

What does ASMR do to your brain?

The popularity of ASMR videos may be due to their potential health benefits. Aside from being a pleasant sensation, many people who watch ASMR videos say it helps reduce symptoms of depression, anxiety and insomnia. The thriving ASMR reddit contains testimonies of people who are thrilled that they can consistently trigger the sensation and its associated benefits by watching ASMR videos when they feel stressed.

Our recent research suggests that these claims are plausible. In a controlled experiment, in which people who experience ASMR watched these videos, they reported feeling much calmer and their heart rates slowed.

The effect was comparable to that found in mindfulness exercises which psychologists recommend, such as interventions in which patients are encouraged to accept emotions rather than suppress them. Survey research suggests that the most common motivation for watching ASMR videos is for the mental health benefit of aiding sleep and reducing stress.

However, one of the obstacles to ASMR as a therapeutic tool is the differing extent to which people experience ASMR. Some people do not experience it at all, and others may only experience it in response to certain triggers, or in certain situations. More research is needed to find out under which conditions ASMR is strongest and most reliable.

At the moment, there is a lack of scientific research explaining the origins of ASMR, although there have been interesting suggestions for possible avenues to explore. Could ASMR be something like the opposite of misophonia, a condition that makes people experience negative reactions to lip smacking, eating or slurping sounds?

Alternatively, feeling a tingling sensation from triggering ASMR sounds could be related to synaesthesia – the ability of some people to experience stimuli in multiple ways, such as associating certain sounds with visual colour.

Despite the popularity of ASMR, the scientific community is only just beginning to recognise it as a worthy phenomenon to study. There is much that we don't know about ASMR, but our early findings suggest it could be an effective tool for people who experience it to reduce stress in the digital age.

21 August 2018

UK teenagers turn to mobile apps to help with mental ill-health

By Dennis Campbell

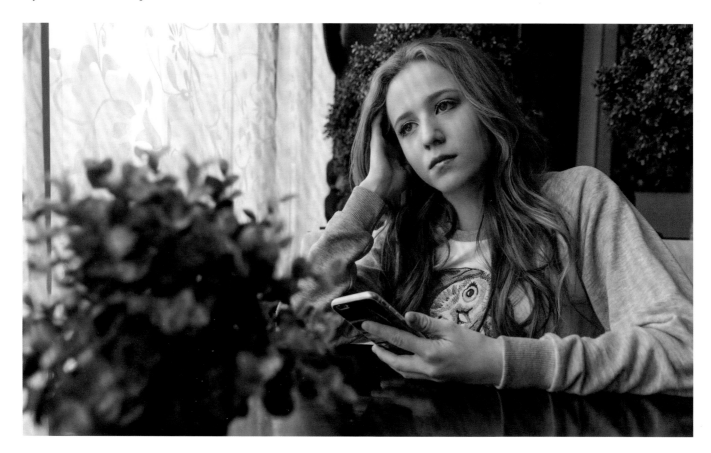

Tens of thousands of young people in Britain who are struggling with their mental health are seeking help online for problems such as anxiety, self-harm and depression.

Soaring numbers of under-18s are turning to apps, online counselling and 'mood diaries' to help them manage and recover from conditions that have left them feeling low, isolated and, in some cases, suicidal.

A generation of young people are attracted by being able to receive fast, personal care and advice using their phone rather than having to wait up to 18 months to be treated by an NHS mental health professional.

The shift comes as ministers brace themselves for publication on Thursday of the first new figures for 13 years showing how common mental heath problems are in the young.

Experts believe they will show a big rise from the one in ten schoolchildren who were identified as having a diagnosable mental health condition when the last research was done in 2005, partly as a result of the emergence of social media and its use in cyberbullying and fuelling feelings of inadequacy The number of under-18s using Kooth, a free online counselling service, has shot up from 20,000 in 2015 to 65,000 last year, and is forecast to rise further to 100,000 this year.

100 NHS clinical commissioning groups across England, more than half the total, have now commissioned the service. It helps young people suffering from anxiety, low mood, poor self-worth or confidence, self-harm and loneliness.

'Young people like the fact they can talk to a counsellor either instantly, or within ten minutes, for up to an hour in the evenings. They love that immediacy,' said Aaron Sefi, the research and evaluation director at XenZone, the company behind Kooth.

'They also love the anonymity involved, because they can sign up without giving their personal details. Plus, they're in control, because they are choosing to contact us rather than being told to do so.'

Its use of video counselling and supportive text messages also help young people feel less alone, he said.

In addition, 123,138 people in the UK downloaded Calm Harm, an NHS-approved app that helps people self-harm less often or not at all, between April 2017 and this month. Of those, 56% were aged between ten and 18 and 82% were girls or women.

'Users tell us that Calm Harm helps with suicidal thoughts and intent,' said Dr Nihara Krause, the consultant clinical psychologist who developed the app. 'Currently 92% of our users, who are mainly female and often aged 15-21, say the urge reduced.'

The app, which launched in 2015, also helps people who have impulse control problems, such as obsessive compulsive disorder, eating disorders and problem drinking, she said.

Calm Harm is among 18 apps that NHS England has endorsed to help tackle mental ill-health.

They also include Blue Ice, which helps young people manage their emotions using a mood diary, techniques to reduce feelings of distress and automatic routing to emergency help numbers if their urges to self-harm continue.

Experts welcomed the trend but warned that online help must complement, not replace, face-to-face appointments with therapists, psychologists and psychiatrists.

'Most young people spend much of their time online, and it can feel easier for them to communicate through messaging and online services than face-to-face,' said Tom Madders, campaigns director at Young Minds, which helps people under 26.

'Evidence-based mental health apps and online support services can be really beneficial in helping young people to look after their own mental health, develop strategies for coping with difficult emotions, and get accessible information and advice when they need it.'

Claire Murdoch, NHS England's national mental health director, said: 'Technology is constantly evolving and young people are usually at the forefront, so it's no surprise increasing numbers are turning to services like these which can certainly play a part, particularly when backed up by face-to-face support.'

The NHS's forthcoming long-term plan, due next month, will 'harness all of the benefits these advancements can bring", she added.

Meanwhile, 37% of the young people referred to NHS child and adolescent mental health services (Camhs) in England last year were refused help, the children's commissioner has revealed.

In an analysis of Camhs care published on Thursday, the children's commissioner for England, Anne Longfield, says that despite promises by politicians and NHS bosses to improve access, 'a vast gap remains between what is provided and what children need'.

While she found improvements in several areas of care, including care for eating disorders, new mothers and under-18s in the criminal justice system, overall 'the current rate of progress is still not good enough for the majority of children who require help but are not receiving it'.

Of more than 338,000 children and young people referred to Camhs last year, 31% were treated within a year. But 37% got no help at all and another 32% were still waiting for treatment to start at the end of the year, she found.

In the UK, Samaritans can be contacted on 116 123.

22 November 2018

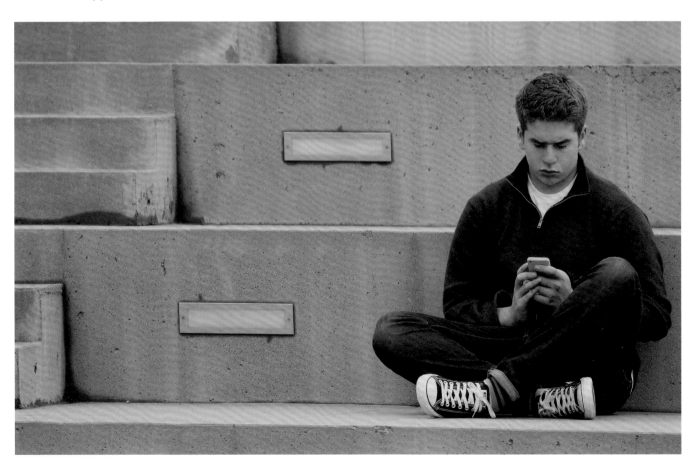

Key facts

⇨ At least two children in every primary school class (based on average class size of 27) are likely to have a diagnosable mental health condition. This rises to three to four students in every class by secondary school age. Around a further six to eight children in each primary school class will be struggling just below this 'unwell' threshold. (pages 3–4)

⇨ A study recently published by Schaefer and colleagues (2017) established that over 80% of participants from their health and development study were found to have a diagnosable mental health condition, from the time of their birth to midlife. This was amongst a representative group of more than 1,000 people studied over a four-decade period. (page 4)

⇨ Nine out of ten people with mental health problems experience stigma and discrimination. (page 7)

⇨ In the last six years the number of working days lost to stress, depression and anxiety has increased by 24%. (page 7)

⇨ 70 million working days are lost each year due to mental ill health, costing Britain annually £70–100 billion. (page 7)

⇨ Since 1981, the proportion of male to female suicides has increased steadily with four in five suicides being male. (page 7)

⇨ The UK has the fourth highest rate of antidepressant prescriptions in Europe at 50 million per year. (page 7)

⇨ A National Centre for Social Research study in 2017 found one in eight (12.8%) five to 19-year-olds had at least one mental disorder at the time of interview. One in 18 (5.5%) preschool children (those aged two to four) were also identified with a mental disorder. (page 11)

⇨ Of the 1.4 million new referrals for talking therapies as part of NHS England's Increasing Access to Talking Therapies (IAPT) programme, 965,000 people began treatment, a 32,000 rise on patient numbers from the year before. (page 12)

⇨ A recent survey carried out by the Association for Teachers and Lecturers (ATL) found that 82% of educators believe children and young people are under more pressure now than they were ten years ago, with 89% considering that testing and exams were the biggest cause. (page 13)

⇨ Childline is a service that provides advice and counselling to anyone under 19 in the UK, and is part of the NSPCC. It delivered over 3,000 counselling sessions online or over the phone on exam stress in 2016/17, which is a 2% increase on what it dealt with in 2015/16 and 11% up on two years ago. (page 14)

⇨ Figures published in 2015 show that NHS spending on children's mental health services in the UK has fallen by 5.4% in real terms since 2010 to £41 million, despite an increase in demand. (page 15)

⇨ Three-quarters of people in the UK have felt 'overwhelmed or unable to cope' at some point in the last year, according to the largest study of its kind. (page 17)

⇨ Young people are most likely to be highly stressed with 83% of 18–24 year-olds saying this compared to 65% of people aged 55 and over. A gender divide also emerged: 81% of women felt this way compared to 67% of men. (page 17)

⇨ More than one in ten children (11%) aged between ten and 15 say they have no one to talk to or wouldn't talk to anyone in school if they feel worried or sad, according to a new survey commissioned by the Mental Health Foundation. (page 18)

⇨ According to Public Health England, 10% of children and young people in England (aged 5–16) have a clinically diagnosable mental health problem. (page 18)

⇨ Figures in a BMA report point to a 9.1 per cent increase in the prevalence of depression between 2015–16 and 2016–17 and a 44 per cent increase in contacts with mental health and learning disability services between 2014–15 and 2016–17. (page 22)

⇨ The number of mental illness overnight beds dropped by 62% in the 20 years to 2009. (page 23)

⇨ There were the equivalent of around 3,200 full-time junior doctors specialising in psychiatry training in September 2009. That number had fallen by around 500, or 15% by September 2017 – the most recent comparable figures. (page 23)

⇨ Recent research published in the *Journal of Affective Disorders* explored how the Bank of England interest rate changes influenced people's mental health. The report found that for each one per cent increase in interest rates, there was a 2.6 per cent increase in the incidence of mental health issues experienced by those heavily indebted. (page 26)

⇨ Since the 'Mind Over Matter' study started in 2008 there were significantly more anti-stigmatising articles (50%) than stigmatising (35%) articles. The remainder of articles were mixed (6%) or neutral (9%). (page 30)

⇨ Levels of self-harm rose by 20% in prisons in 2018, and at least nine out of ten prisoners has at least one mental health problem. (page 34)

⇨ The number of under-18s using Kooth, a free online counselling service, has shot up from 20,000 in 2015 to 65,000 last year, and is forecast to rise further to 100,000 this year. (page 38)

⇨ Of more than 338,000 children and young people referred to Camhs last year, 31% were treated within a year. But 37% got no help at all and another 32% were still waiting for treatment to start at the end of the year. (page 39)

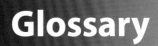

Anxiety

Anxiety can be described as a feeling of fear, apprehension, tension and/or stress. Most people experience anxiety from time to time and this is a perfectly normal response to stress. However, some individuals suffer from anxiety disorders which cause them to experience symptoms such as intense, persistent fear or nervousness, panic attacks and hyperventilation.

ASMR

Autonomous Sensory Meridian Response - is an experience characterized by a tingling sensation on the skin that typically begins on the scalp and moves down the back of the neck and upper spine. Similar to the sensation of having 'goosebumps'.

Bipolar disorder

Previously called manic depression, this illness is characterised by mood swings where periods of severe depression are balanced by periods of elation and overactivity (mania).

Cognitive behavioural therapy (CBT)

A psychological treatment which assumes that behavioural and emotional reactions are learned over a long period. A cognitive therapist will seek to identify the source of emotional problems and develop techniques to overcome them.

Depression

Someone is said to be significantly depressed, or suffering from depression, when feelings of sadness or misery don't go away quickly and are so bad that they interfere with everyday life. Symptoms can also include low self-esteem and a lack of motivation.

Mental health/well-being

Everyone has 'mental health'. It includes our emotional, psychological and social well-being. It affects how we think, feel, and act. It also helps determine how we handle stress, relate to others, and make choices. Mental health is important at every stage of life, from childhood and adolescence through adulthood.

Mindfulness

Mind-bod- based training that uses meditation, breathing and yoga techniques to help you focus on your thoughts and feelings. Mindfulness helps you manage your thoughts and feelings better, instead of being overwhelmed by them.

Obsessive compulsive disorder (OCD)

Obsessive compulsive disorder (OCD) is a common mental health condition in which a person has obsessive thoughts and compulsive behaviours. It affects men, women and children, and can develop at any age. Some people develop the condition early, often around puberty, but it typically develops during early adulthood.

Personality disorder

Personality disorder is a type of mental health problem where your attitudes, beliefs and behaviours that can cause longstanding problems. There are several different categories and types of personality disorder, but most people who are diagnosed with a particular personality disorder don't fit any single category very clearly or consistently. Also, the term 'personality disorder' can sound very judgemental. Because of this it is a particularly controversial diagnosis. Some psychiatrists disagree with using it.

Post-Traumatic Stress Disorder (PTSD)

PTSD is a psychological response to an intensely traumatic event. It is commonly observed in members of the armed forces and has been known by different names at different times in history: during the First World War, for example, it was known as 'shell shock'.

Psychiatrist

A medical doctor who specialises in diagnosing and treating mental disorders. This is different from a psychologist, who is a professional or academic (not necessarily a doctor) specialising in understanding the human mind, thought and human behaviour.

Psychosis

A mental state in which the perception of reality is distorted.

Schizophrenia

Disorder characterised by hallucinations, paranoid delusions and abnormal thought patterns.

Assignments

Brainstorming

⇨ In small groups, discuss what you know about mental health and mental illness. Consider the following points:

- What is mental health?

- Why is being aware of and looking after your mental health so important?

- Talk about how you look after your own mental health.

- Do you think physical health can affect mental health and vice versa?

- How would you try to support a friend who was struggling with their mental health?

Research

⇨ Read the article on page 6 about media guidelines for reporting on mental health issues. Conduct an online search for recent news stories from different sources which refer to mental illness. Try to find one article which adheres to current guidelines and one which doesn't. Examine the contrast in tone, attitude and language used in each piece and discuss in groups.

⇨ Visit Mind's website: www.mind.org.uk. What are the aims of this organisation? What support do they offer for people suffering from mental health problems? Write a short review of the site, including how accessible you feel the information is and how easy you find the site to use.

⇨ Research mental health charities and support groups in your local area and then think about how you might promote them in your community. Write some notes then feedback to your class.

⇨ Look at the infographic *Mental Health in the UK : The big picture* (page 7) – how do you think this overview of the UK compares with other similar countries across the globe? Choose another country to research, compare and contrast their mental health statistics with the UK's.

Design

⇨ Design a poster to raise awareness for a lesser known mental health condition. Think about where would be the most effective places to display your poster.

⇨ Design an app aimed at helping people struggling with a mental illness. Think about what your app will be called, what it will do and the problems it will address. Produce some sketches and write some ideas about how you would make your app inclusive and appealing to a broad demographic.

⇨ Choose one of the articles in this book and create an illustration to highlight the key themes/message of your chosen article.

⇨ Design a website that will give parents information about mental wellbeing in young people. Think about the kind of information they might need and give your site a name and design a logo.

Oral

⇨ Role-play a situation in which one of you is an employer looking to fill a vacancy within your company and the other is someone applying for the job who is well qualified for the job but suffers from a mental illness, such as bipolar disorder. Put yourself in that person's position and think carefully about what kind of questions and concerns you might have. Take it in turns to play the role of the employer and the job-seeker.

⇨ 'Social media, exam stress and gaming addictions are the biggest threats to young people's mental health today.' Debate this motion as a class, with one group arguing in favour and the other against.

Reading/writing

⇨ Write a diary entry from the point of view of someone who suffers from a mental illness such as depression. Imagine how they would feel and what challenges they could face in their day-to-day life. You may need to do further research into the mental illness you have chosen.

⇨ Read the article *These black women felt excluded by mainstream mental health charities – so they started thier own* (pages 24–25). Can you identify any gaps in your local community support networks where a group of people or a particular mental health condition are under-represented? If so, explore how you would go about setting up a charity or a support group to address the un-met mental health needs in your local area.

⇨ Think about someone in the public eye who has spoken out about their own personal mental health issues. Write a short biography of that person and describe what you admire/find inspirational about them.

⇨ Visit some online newspaper archives and find an old news story referring to mental illness that uses out-dated terminology that stigmatises mental heath problems Now, look at the article about reporting on mental health (page 6) and rewite the article according to today's media guidelines.

Acknowledgements

The publisher is grateful for permission to reproduce the material in this book. While every care has been taken to trace and acknowledge copyright, the publisher tenders its apology for any accidental infringement or where copyright has proved untraceable. The publisher would be pleased to come to a suitable arrangement in any such case with the rightful owner.

Images

All images courtesy of iStock except pages 1, 4, 17, 30, 36, 37, 38, 39: Pixabay. 2, 8, 9, 12, 13, 15, 16, 24, 25, 26, 28, 29, 32, 35: Unsplash. 31: Rawpixel.

Icons

Icons on page 7 were made by catkuro, Freepik, Good Ware, Maxim Basinski, OCHA, Plainicon, Smashicons and Those Icons; all from www.flaticon.com.

Icons on page 18 were made by pixelperfect and Freepik, from www.flaticon.com.

Illustrations

Don Hatcher: pages 14 & 33. Simon Kneebone: pages 5 & 34. Angelo Madrid: pages 19 & 22.

Additional acknowledgements

With thanks to the Independence team: Shelley Baldry, Tina Brand, Danielle Lobban, Jackie Staines and Jan Sunderland.

Tracy Biram

Cambridge, January 2019